THE TIM

CALM SUTRA
THE ART OF RELAXATION

DR. DILIP NADKARNI

Calm Sutra: The Art of Relaxation
Book copyright © 2008, Bennett, Coleman & Co., Ltd.

First Edition 2008

Published by
Ravi Dhariwal for the proprietors,
Bennett, Coleman & Co. Ltd.,
New Delhi

All Rights Reserved.
No part of this work may be reproduced or used in any form or by any means (graphic, electronic, mechanical, photocopying, recording, tape, web distribution, information storage and retrieval systems or otherwise) without prior written permission of the publisher.

Disclaimer:
BCCL does not represent or endorse accuracy or reliability of any content provided in the Book and any reliance upon such content shall be at the reader's sole risk. Such content as provided in this Book does not represent the views of BCCL or its advertisers or sponsors. Due care and diligence has been taken while editing and printing the Book, neither the Publisher nor the Printer of the Book hold any responsibility for any mistake that may have crept in inadvertently. BCCL will be free from any liability for damages and losses of any nature arising from or related to the content. All disputes are subject to the jurisdiction of competent courts in Delhi.

ISBN 978-81-89906-25-2

Editorial Team	: Madhulita Mohanty, Jai Narayan Ram
Design	: Subhasish Munshi, Jitender Kumar
Printed And Bound By	: Paras Offset (P) Ltd.
Price	: Rs.150/-

Contents

- Introduction to Calm Sutra 5
- Acknowledgements 9
- What is Calm Sutra? 11
- Why Stress on Calm Sutra? 13
- What are Stressors? 19
- Ill Effects of Stress 23
- Can Stress be Helpful? 31
- The Calm Sutra Stress Busters 35
- Proactive Attitude 41
- Being in the Present 49
- Deep Breathing 53
- Progressive Muscle Relaxation 63
- The Postures of Calm Sutra 73
- Meditation 81
- Meditative Eating 93
- Visualization, in your Personal Theatre 99
- Positive Affirmations 107
- Laughter 115

CALM SUTRA : THE ART OF RELAXATION

- ❖ Put Your Worries to Sleep 119
- ❖ Massage 125
- ❖ Calm Sutra of Sex 133
- ❖ Music 139
- ❖ Dance Away your Blues .149
- ❖ Exercise: A potent Stress Buster 155
- ❖ Stretching 163
- ❖ Weight Training 168
- ❖ Aerobic Exercise 173
- ❖ Walking Away from Stress 181
- ❖ Running to De-Stress 189
- ❖ Swimming 195
- ❖ Table Tennis 200
- ❖ Golf 205
- ❖ Epilogue 213
- ❖ The Calm Sutra Workshop (CSW) 214
- ❖ About the Author 215

Introduction to Calm Sutra

As I was completing an arthroscopic surgery, I announced to my anaesthetist, that I was taking a break and pushing off to Goa for a week.

"With family or only with your wife for a monsoon honeymoon", she asked.

"Neither," I said. "I am going alone. In fact it is to work on a book. The book will be titled as Calm Sutra."

"Wow, I knew orthopaedic surgeons thought themselves to be God, but Sex God is new." She exclaimed.

"C.A.L.M. S.U.T.R.A." I spelt it out for her. "Calm Sutra, the Art of Relaxation. The book will deal with stress management", I added, looking for approval, appreciation and encouragement. After all an anaesthetist is not only a closely working colleague but often a good sounding board for a surgeon.

"Thank God," she took off; "we all need it, having to work with orthopaedic surgeons. I am sure the book will help your wife considering that she has to work and live with an orthopaedic surgeon. But who has given you the license to write a book on stress management? Orthopaedic surgeons should write a book on stress creation, since you are so good at it." She went on and on....

I followed one of the key principles of

> Those who can, they do. Those who can't, they teach.
>
> *Anonymous*

Calm Sutra: Take a Calm Pause. Let Go. Agree to Disagree.

As an orthopaedic surgeon, I am used to being taunted at; being the butt of jokes and not being credited with much brains or knowledge of general medicine.

You must have heard some classic ones on orthopaedic surgeons; like this one, which is a favourite of all anaesthetists:

"What is the difference between God and an orthopaedic surgeon?"

"Well, God does not think he is an orthopaedic surgeon!"

Or, "What's the difference between a rhino and an orthopaedic surgeon?"

"One is a thick skinned, pea brained, short sighted guy who charges excessively for no rhyme or reason. And the other one is a rhino!

I am told rhinos took serious objection to being compared with orthopaedic surgeons.

GENESIS OF CALM SUTRA

A few years ago I wrote a book, titled *REAL Fitness*. REAL is a mnemonic where R stands for Relaxation, E for Exercise, A for Attitude and L for Laughter. Having read the book, a few corporate bodies invited me to conduct sessions on fitness and stress management for their executives. Though rated highly by the audience and enjoyed by me, these sessions became less frequent due to my surgical commitments.

Recently, I met a good friend Dr R K Sanghavi, a medical advisor to top pharmaceutical companies, at the Bombay Presidency Golf Club. My golf game was rained out and I got chatting with him. Knowing that he was not a golfer, I enquired about the purpose of his visit to our club. He said that he was conducting a training session for a pharmaceutical company, Svizera Healthcare, in the banquet hall of our golf club. He felt that his delegates needed a diversion from the heavy academic training they were subjected to.

I suggested that I could do a relaxation session for them with meditation, music, exercises, postural tips and a round of golf

INTRODUCTION TO CALM SUTRA

thrown in. He called up Mr. Shailesh Patil, the general manager of Svizera, and the idea was welcomed. The module titled 'Calm Sutra, the Art of Relaxation' was announced.

So that day, instead of hitting golf balls, I interacted with 20 delegates from the pharma company. We spoke, we stretched, we sang, we meditated; we relaxed and generally had a ball. The appreciation I got from the delegates of Svizera Healthcare, spurred me to revive and update the module on relaxation and stress management. Why not have this training module in a book form, I asked myself. It woke up the dormant writer in me. The hotel and flights to Goa were booked and Calm Sutra was conceived.

In the case of Calm Sutra, the title came first and then the book followed. It is quite similar to having a baby because you liked a particular name.

WHY GOA?

There is no better place in the world to think, write or live Calm Sutra. Goa, in all languages, means 'to chill out'. Goa emanates the essence of Calm Sutra with the idyllic beaches, the swaying palms, the friendly people, the food, the drink, the music, the siestas and of course, the carnival. When I decided to take a break, to work on the book, there was no debate on the destination.

THE PURPOSE OF CALM SUTRA

Well, Calm Sutra is a book for myself. It is a manual for me to follow, to understand and ward off stress; and be happy.

To quote Khalil Gibran:

To the prophet, on the day of his departure, Almitra the seeress said, Blessed be this day and this place and your spirit that has spoken. And he answered, *Was it I who spoke? Was I not also a listener?*

A wise man said to a fat man, "If you want to lose weight and maintain it, start lecturing on fitness".

Here I am writing the Calm Sutra so that I am the first reader and a committed follower of relaxed, stress-free living. At no time do I want people to witness behaviour from me, which would prompt them to say, "Are you really the author of Calm Sutra?"

If I can transmit relaxation and happiness to my family, friends and patients it would be a great bonus. If you accept my invitation to visit the fascinating world of Calm Sutra, my mission is accomplished.

AM I A GURU?

Definitely not. To be frank, I think I am quite spiritually challenged.

But I have a vision of myself. While practising creative visualization, I have seen myself as Baba Calm Dev, a relaxed and happy man. Baba is a leader in his chosen profession and yet has enough time for his family and friends. He is proactive, healthy and cheerful; he exercises, meditates, sings and laughs, goes on vacations, and of course plays golf!

You will keep hearing from Baba Calm Dev from time to time. His attempt at humour is itself comic at times and needs a little patience, but let me assure you, he means well.

Welcome to Calm Sutra.

Acknowledgements

I would like to acknowledge the role of my parents, Geeta and Vasant Nadkarni, for all that they have done for me. I thank them for providing me a rich upbringing full of sports, music, academics and fun.

My wife Rashmi needs to be awarded for putting up with me and my sense of humour, and yet escaping unscathed. This book would not have been possible without her love and support.

Cheers to my children Nishad and Rishab who are quite chilled-out characters, who could add a chapter or two to Calm Sutra.

I thank all my teachers who have provided me with unparalleled inputs making this book possible.

A special thanks to my friends who have spent real quality time with me and enriched my life.

A very proactive thank you to my co-golfers for all the testing time they give me, which gives me a chance to practice and live "Calm Sutra".

A big thank you my friend Dr Bharat Shah, eminent psychiatrist and former president of Bombay Psychiatry Society for his invaluable inputs on the topic of stress.

Please consult your physician before starting any physical activity mentioned in this book.

What is Calm Sutra?

CHAPTER 1

Calm Sutra is a way of life that one can adopt to be relaxed, calm, healthy and happy. As the writer and the first reader of Calm Sutra, I try to live my life, the Calm Sutra way. As I continue to live by the tenets of Calm Sutra, I have begun to notice lower levels of stress in my life. I feel I am assaying to live up to my potential with increased productivity and success. The Happiness Quotient seems to improve, as I find more reasons to be happy. And sometimes even for no apparent reason, I am happy.

PRINCIPLES OF CALM SUTRA: AA

Calm Sutra essentially revolves around two main principles: **Awareness** and **Action**, both of which are intrinsically related and dependant on each other. Awareness of our body is vital towards understanding the various processes and needs that arise within the system. This comes with a certain degree of sensitivity and deep understanding of our self.

Awareness directs the individual to take proactive action, in the desired direction, wherever needed. This is the basis of good health. For example, an awareness of our posture helps us to maintain a sound body alignment. Again, awareness of our breathing techniques can lead us to adopt appropriate deep breathing techniques that could be the cure for a lot of diseases. Awareness of thought can help us streamline our thoughts

> Calm Sutra, yes, it is fun intended all the way.
> *Baba Calm Dev*

and take concerted action. This is especially true for situations that are stressful. In a nutshell, awareness helps us enjoy life better since it brings with it a deep sense of consciousness, acknowledgement, and alertness and above all heightens responsiveness of the individual to his environment. Therefore, being aware is one of the most important prerequisites in our quest for happiness and fulfillment.

The other vital principle that forms the basis of Calm Sutra is the action principle. This is a self-explanatory principle and depends completely on correct assessment and appraisal of the situation. It also depends on a certain attitude. We call it the proactive attitude and as all attitudes are wont to do; this proactive attitude too determines our behaviour towards a certain event or individual. Attitudes are based on information and hence the awareness principle needs to be at its heightened best so as to produce evaluations that are precise and well grounded.

So, we see that with deep awareness and understanding an individual's reaction could be more appropriate. It would help him stay calm in the face of stress, as well as understand and make correct assessment of the situation. This interplay between awareness and action is the crux of Calm Sutra.

The book seeks to heighten the awareness and action potentials in an individual through a gamut of exercises and techniques. It aims to make an individual derive pleasure from the little things in life; live life as it is - composed of little moments and experiences.

> Calm Sutra essentially revolves around 2 principles: **Awareness** and **Action** — the **AA** of Calm Sutra.

CHAPTER 2

Why Stress on Calm Sutra?

STRESS: AN INTRODUCTION

Individual life is fraught with stress and there is rarely a person who does not encounter stress at some point in his life. Stress really has no age or time bar and individual lifestyles and ineffective coping patterns are forcing a lot of medical practitioners to sit up and take notice. Innumerable lifestyle diseases have their genesis in stress levels within the individual. In fact, children too are falling prey to increasing levels of stress. Therefore, to correctly interpret the Calm Sutra, let us begin with getting a fair understanding of stress, the effect it has on us and individual efforts at dealing with stress.

The term stress has many definitions. However, in psychological terms, we describe stress as an internal state that can be caused by physical demands on the body (like disease, especially debilitating ones; extremities in temperature; high-powered exercise and the likes). Other causal factors would be demands made by the physical and social environment.

UNDERSTANDING THE GENESIS OF STRESS

The physical, environmental and social factors that induce feelings of discomfort at the physiological and psychological level are

> Tension is who you think you should be. Relaxation is who you are.
> *Chinese Proverb*

called stressors and they promote feelings of great inadequacy and inability to cope. Hence stressors, in absolute commonplace parlance can be explained as events or situations that trigger a stress response.

Stressors are completely dependant on individual capacity to cope adequately and this is where variations come in. A single stressor is likely to induce discomfort in one individual, in more varying degrees than another. Similarly, the same individual may react differently to the same stressor at different points of his life. Hence, individual differences or variations are of utmost importance in an analysis of stress.

It would be pertinent to mention in the course of this chapter that all changes, even positive ones, bring in some amount of stress. Till such time an individual can cope, the stress is considered 'optimal'. More than that is 'distress' and this is where individual capacities are tested.

Stress brings with it a number of effects. Some immediate, which if maintained, go into long term behavioural, physiological, emotional and cognitive manifestations. Physical manifestations would include accelerating levels of blood pressure, increase in heart beat rate, breathlessness, frequent bowel movements, nausea, fatigue, incapacity to think properly etc. Over a sustained period of time, these may lead to cardiac diseases, high BP, digestive problems, ulcers, insomnia chronic fatigue and even hair loss.

The psychological manifestations would include limited cognitive capacities and behavioural problems, especially anxiety-based disorders, such as obsessive compulsive disorders, phobias, panic attacks, social anxiety, depression, memory loss, inability to control anger, frustration, and an overall lack of concentration in almost all areas of life.

STRESSORS AND WHAT THEY DO TO THE BODY

Walter Cannon in 1932 established the existence of a gamut of responses which he collectively termed as a **Flight-or-Fight Response**. Stressors actually induce certain emotions which in turn

CHAPTER 2 : WHY STRESS ON CALM SUTRA?

affect the bodily states. Increased activity in the parasympathetic nervous system leads to a pattern of activity that equips the body to fight the emergency situation by either adopting the flight response or by adopting the fright response.

Emotional states, especially in case of fear and anger, cause heartbeat rates to increase, blood vessels and pupils to dilate. There is muscular preparedness, blood flow is available more to the muscles and redirected from the skin so as to minimize blood loss if one is injured, blood sugar is mobilized from the liver, hormones like epinephrine and nor epinephrine are released from the adrenal gland. All these improve an individual's preparedness to survive stressful situations.

As stated earlier, stress impairs the cognitive capacities of the individual and often, wrong decisions are taken which may have untold consequences on the life and relationships of the individual.

In day to day life, the flight or fright response usually occurs in face of unexpected crisis which is not of a very high intensity. So, in a way these reactions are considered 'normal'. Most of the situations faced by individuals require a more proactive approach that encourages awareness and action. This is where Calm Sutra might prove to be useful, especially for those in high capacity positions/situations which are often hot stress beds.

THE PATH TO BURNOUT

Hans Selye, regarded as the father of stress analysis, took a slightly different approach from Cannon. He identified a general response and named it "General Adaptation Syndrome". Selye identified that when pushed to extremes, animals react in three stages:

First, in the **Alarm Phase**, they react to the stressor, with a typical release of the stress hormones. This is a stage of shock with the basic stress hormones coming into play.

Next, is the **Resistance Phase** or the adaptation phase where the animals try to cope with stress. As the stress increases, the resistance to the stressor also increases as the animal adapts to it. This phase lasts for as long as the animal could carry on coping with the stress.

Translated to human behaviour, this is the phase where the stressed person is in a constant state of worry. He often stops living in the present moment. He is either worrying about the future or brooding over the past. There is a constant mental chatter or the Brownian movement of thought, which triggers off a lot of health problems.

Finally, once resistance was exhausted, the animal entered the **Exhaustion Phase**, and resistance declined substantially.

In the business environment, this **exhaustion** is seen as a "**burnout**". The classic example comes from the share market trading area. Life in the stock market is stressful to say the least. Traders learn to adapt or cope with the stressful ups and downs of the stock market, but a prolonged exposure to such stresses leaves them exhausted.

Some of the signs of burn out include chronic fatigue, emotional exhaustion, self-criticism, cynicism and feeling of helplessness. There could be frank physical manifestations like frequent headaches, gastrointestinal disturbances, weight loss or gain and other psychosomatic conditions attributed to stress.

Burn outs are also seen in the sports arena. Young achievers struggle hard to reach a high level of competence in sports. They motivate themselves, work on their fitness, practice hours on end, play the circuit all over the world and expose themselves to a lot of pressure. A day comes when they cannot take it anymore and simply burn out.

WHO SUCCUMBS TO STRESS?

For people to become "stressed" there are two pre-requisites:

Firstly, they must feel threatened by the situation.

Secondly, they must feel that they are not capable or not resourceful enough to meet the threat.

A person gets stressed when he is buying a house. He is afraid that the loan is too much. He feels that it will upset his life by making him bankrupt. He worries about the future, as to what will happen to his wife and family. The loan is perceived as a threat.

CHAPTER 2 : WHY STRESS ON CALM SUTRA?

For stress to precipitate, threat alone is not enough. He has to presume that he is incapable of paying back the loan. He has to feel that his business is not resourceful enough to generate the installments, only then stress will happen. If he thinks coolly and plans proactively about the resources and ways to pay back the loan, the stress will be less.

These perceived threats arising from our thought process trigger the hormonal fight-or-flight response, with all of its negative consequences.

THOUGHT FOR THE DAY

'Thought for the day' is a myth because research tells us that on an average a human being has close to 60,000 thoughts everyday. So a single thought in a day is really impossible.

Most of these thoughts that pass through the mind are unstructured, chaotic and lack cohesion. They are often responsible for creating a stressful situation and bringing with them several maladies. They take us away from the moment and leave us confused.

When these uncluttered thoughts dominate our mind, it brings on stress and lets loose an entire gamut of bodily reactions. Hormones get released, behavioural and facial gestures change, the heart beat rates accelerate, blood pressure levels go upwards, breathing becomes shallower and the person loses his sleep and appetite. All of this can be avoided with certain techniques, most of which will be explored in the chapters that are to follow. However, it must be kept in mind that the individual and his will are the most powerful tools and it is he alone who can obstruct the intrusion of such random stressful thoughts that are a peril to good life and health.

MY TRYST WITH STRESS

As an orthopaedic surgeon, I encounter stress in many forms. I see acute stress in patients coming in the operation theatre. They are apprehensive about the operation, the anaesthesia, the final outcome, costs of hospitalization etc.

I see chronic stress presenting itself with bad posture, backache, neck pains, knee pains and many other vague but genuine complaints. Stressed patients usually show a delay in recovery after surgery. Though many orthopaedic surgeons may not like to show it, there is stress at work. The stress could range from patient bleeding on table, poor surgical outcome, anaesthesia complications, to delays in operation schedules and dissatisfied patients.

As a person, I do not claim to have survived the holocaust or fought a war, but by the virtue of being married, qualifies me to say something about stress!

In the next chapter we shall try and identify the common stressors, which elicit the stress response.

> Stress, today's key 'debilitator', is basically an internal response from our mind and body to unpleasant situations and events.
>
> It is a reaction to "stressors" that disturb our natural physical, emotional or mental balance.

What are Stressors?

CHAPTER 3

Stress as a subject of research received momentum in the 1950s and was used as a term to explain all kinds of pressures that an individual experienced. It also included within its ambit behavioural manifestations resulting from these pressures. Collectively, the term given to these pressures are stressors. So in a very technical sense, any stimulus that produces stress is called a **stressor**. A stressor may be in the form of an individual, event or a feeling.

Stressors are present all around us. It would not be an exaggeration to say that they are strewn like landmines; some are cleverly concealed while others, not so well disguised. Often stressors have a way of coming on without warning and it is imperative that one knows how to identify and deal with them, so as not to upset the rhythm of life, health and happiness too much.

> Stresspassers will be prosecuted.
> *Baba Calm Dev*

STRESSORS: A CLASSIFICATION
Major and Minor Stressors

Stressors can be classified into two types: major and minor. As the term denotes, **major stressors** are the ones that cause acute stress. The death of a spouse, separation, failing in an examination, loss in business etc. are examples of major stressors.

Minor stressors would include those events that do not produce stress in high magnitudes. However, minor stressors, by sheer dint of recurrence in a person's life over an extended period of time may lead to chronic stress. This can be extremely non conducive to mental and physical health in the long run. Working with unreasonable deadlines, trying to achieve impossible targets, constant bickering with in-laws, irrational demands by spouse, pollution etc can take a heavy toll on a person.

Dr Prabodh Karnik, an eminent ear surgeon, emphasizes the role of noise as a potent stressor. According to him, noise produces a discordant effect on the mind and can in many cases affect hearing capacities. Noise in this case is a minor stressor; however, over a certain period of time, it can become a chronic stressor with enough potential to cause damage. Thus, the point to be understood is that minor stressors work stealthily and are often recognized after the damage has been done.

STRESSORS: INTRINSIC AND EXTRINSIC

All stressors need not be **extrinsic** or environmental. They can also be **intrinsic**, that is arising from within the individual. Stress induced as a result of poor health, insecurity or poor self esteem are examples of intrinsic stressors. Whatever be the source of stress, it is imperative that an individual recognizes his state and identifies factors that are affecting this condition. Concerted efforts can only pay off if the cause is identified correctly.

IMPACT OF STRESSORS: A FUNCTION OF CHANGING VARIABLES

Stressors differ in their impact. So, it is not at all uncommon to see the same individual reacting to the same stressor differently at different points of time. So, what are the variables that alter the impact of stressors on the individual?

Age

The age of the individual is a crucial determinant in the way he handles stress. The same stressors have different impacts on persons of different ages. For example, a death of a parent is a much greater stressor for a child than it is for a middle aged person. The stressors encountered by teenagers are quite different from that of a corporate person. Senior citizens react to stressors in their own way that is determined by their age and life experiences.

Gender
Different stressors may affect genders differently. In one study, work stress was associated with a higher risk for heart disease in men. In women, marital discord and disharmony produced more stress which was manifested in heart diseases and other diseases.

COMMON ACUTE STRESSORS
- Death of a spouse or loss of loved ones
- Marital discord leading to divorce and separation
- Personal injury or illness
- Marriage, especially if one is not ready for it
- Loss of a job, even retirement
- Pregnancy, also miscarriages and infertility problems
- Monetary losses, leading to changes in one's financial state

MINOR STRESSORS
At the Workplace
- Novelty of the situation: meeting new clients, new partners, colleagues or staff
- New ventures or projects, especially the challenging ones
- Deadlines or time-related pressures
- Excessive work, resulting in working overtime
- Professional rivalry and competition; bullying bosses and hostile co-workers
- Excessive demands from clients
- Generating new clients or more business for the company

At Home
- Incompatibility with a family member leading to conflicts and tensions

- Family demands on your time and attention
- Marital tensions and conflicts
- Financial pressures
- Illness in the family

STRESSORS PRESENT IN THE ENVIRONMENT
- Traffic jams and delays
- Pollution
- Noise
- Threat of war, political unrest, earthquakes, fires, flooding, riots etc

CALM SUTRA TEACHES US TWO THINGS REGARDING STRESSORS

1) Build **Awareness**　　2)　Take anti-stress **Action**

With regular practice of the basic tenets of Calm Sutra, i.e. awareness, pro-activity, living life with a positive attitude and having the ability to live in the moment, we can learn to identify the situations that produce stress and thereby opt for certain therapeutic processes to handle the situation in the most effective way. Techniques like relaxation, meditation, deep breathing and of course playing golf can be of huge help to a person who wants to bring down his stress levels. These measures help in absorbing the impact of the stressor and keep the individual on the path of good mental and physical health.

> Stressors are unpleasant situations, strewn all around us like landmines. Stress happens when we step on them and get hurt.

CHAPTER 4

Ill Effects of Stress

"It is not the curry but the hurry and worry which causes the stomach ulcer." I remember the thundering voice of my medicine professor telling us, so as he tried to explain the link between mental stress and stomach ulcers.

The medical fraternity has worked around this belief for a long time that stress and physical ailments are inter related. In fact, this has spanned an entire body of work. **Psycho-somatic disorder** was the term used to describe all ailments that seemed to have a deep underlying psychological basis.

In the past, people were told by their doctors to go to spas or seaside resorts when they were ill. This was especially true in case of women as medical judgments and diagnostics were quite gendered. Stress, worry and high-strung emotions were held responsible for a host of ailments and prescriptions often extended to advices for people to take vacations, especially to places where the individual is far removed from his immediate stressful environment.

That stress may be a precursor to a host of maladies started losing ground in the nineteenth century. With better technology, research and empirical evidence, more and more concrete causes of medical illnesses were explored. Physical infirmities were looked at more minutely and with increased knowledge and diagnostic tools available, medical know how expanded. Stress was not

> The necklace of stress is studded with diseases, with death as the pendant.
> *Baba Calm Dev*

recognized as important.

However, in the recent past medical research seems to have turned a full circle. Many scientists and researchers have been rediscovering the links between the stress and physical maladies and disorders. There is enough scientific evidence to prove that stress can be a precipitating cause for not only behavioural problems but also for more serious health issues. Stress does not affect the body in parts; rather it induces discomfort on the whole human system. Hence, there is a huge amount of importance given to stress in modern treatment discourses.

THE MIND AND BODY CONNECTION

Don't let your mind bully your body into believing it must carry the burden of its worries. — Astrid Alauda

Before I present to you a menu card of all the health problems stress can usher in, we need to understand the basic mechanism by which stress induces illness or psycho-somatic diseases.

The **hypothalamic-pituitary-adrenal axis (HPA axis)** connects the mind and body and are the most important constituents that come into play whenever an individual experiences stress. The mind sends messages to the hypothalamus, a hollow, funnel-shaped part of the brain. The hypothalamus activates the pituitary gland, a pea-shaped structure located below the hypothalamus. The pituitary gland is the gland that produces hormones. The pituitary gland stimulates the adrenal or suprarenal glands, which are small, paired, pyramidal organs located at the top of each kidney. The supra renal glands are the ones, which secrete the havoc-creating stress hormones.

The fine interactions between these three organs constitute the HPA axis, a major part of the neuro-hormonal system that controls reactions to stress. It also regulates other body processes like digestion, the immune system, moods, sexuality and the metabolic rate.

All species, from humans to the most ancient organisms share components of the HPA axis. It is the basis for a process which links

CHAPTER 4 : ILL EFFECTS OF STRESS

the brain, the endocrine glands and their hormones. This HPA axis further simplifies Selye's General Adaptation Syndrome theory and it does provide an explanation of psycho-somatic disorders.

STRESS AND DISEASE

The link between stress and disease, especially heart disease is well established. High stress levels lead to a release of stress hormones which accelerate our **heart rate and blood pressure**, putting tension on the arteries. This invariably causes damage to them. As the body deals with this damage, artery walls scar and thicken, which can reduce the supply of blood and oxygen to the heart.

In addition, stress hormones accelerate the heart to increase the blood supply to muscles; blood vessels, however, in the heart may have become so narrow that not enough blood reaches the heart to meet these increased physical demands. This can cause a heart attack.

Stress has also been found to damage the **immune system**, which explains why we catch more colds when we are stressed. It may intensify symptoms in diseases that have an auto-immune component, such as rheumatoid arthritis. It also seems to affect headaches and irritable bowel syndrome, and there are now suggestions of links between stress and cancer.

STRESS AND THE IMMUNE SYSTEM

When you are stressed, the HPA axis is activated and a cascade of hormones is released from the pituitary and adrenal glands. These hormones lead to an increase in the levels of cortisol.

Cortisol is the major steroid hormone produced by our bodies to help us get through stressful situations. Cortisol is closely related to the compound cortisone, which is widely used as an anti-inflammatory drug in creams to treat rashes and in nasal sprays to treat sinusitis and asthma. Cortisol and cortisone basically suppress the immune system and tone down inflammation within the body. In situations of chronic stress your immune cells are less able to respond to an invader like a bacteria or a virus.

This theory explains lower immunity in groups like medical students undergoing exam stress, military troops undergoing extremely grueling physical stress, and couples subjected to marital stress. People in these situations show a prolonged healing time, a decreased ability of their immune systems to respond to vaccination and an increased susceptibility to viral infections like the common cold.

Recent research has found that HIV-infected men with high stress levels progress more rapidly to AIDS when compared to those with lower stress levels. Some evidence suggests that chronic stress triggers an over-production of certain immune factors called cytokines, which in excess levels can have very damaging effects. In fact, the presence of cytokines may partly explain the association between chronic stress and a number of diseases, including heart disease.

STRESS AND PHYSICAL AILMENTS
Heart Disease
Cardiologists will soon be celebrating World Stress Day, considering the increase in the number of patients suffering from stress. Stress is known to precipitate high blood pressure or hypertension. The stress hormones constrict the arteries of the heart and can lead to heart attacks. Stress causes blood to become stickier, increasing the likelihood of an artery-clogging blood clot. Stress appears to impair the clearance of fat molecules in the body, raising blood-cholesterol levels, at least temporarily. In other words, stress is bad news for your heart.

Hypertension and Stroke
Stroke is a sequel to uncontrolled high blood pressure. Hypertension is often precipitated by stress and can cause bleeding in the brain causing a stroke. One survey revealed that men who had a more intense response to stress were more likely to have strokes than those who did not report such distress.

Cancer

Some animal studies suggest that lack of control over stress had negative effects on the immune function and contributed to growth of tumors that are carcinogenic in nature. Although stress reduction techniques have no effect on survival rates, studies show that they are very helpful in improving a cancer patient's quality of life.

Gastrointestinal Problems

The gut and the brain have a close relationship. Many disorders of the digestive system are due to what eats you rather than what you eat. Prolonged stress can disrupt the function of the gastrointestinal tract. The stomach and duodenum can be victim of excessive acid secretion leading to ulcers and the large intestine can be irritated causing diarrhea or constipation. In fact, some experts estimate that stress is the key player in 30 to 60 per cent of peptic ulcer cases.

Irritable bowel syndrome is strongly related to stress. In this condition, the abdomen is bloated and the patient experiences cramping and alternating periods of constipation and diarrhea.

Diabetes

Stress may be one of the biggest factors causing uncontrolled presence of sugar in the blood stream. Chronic stress has been blamed for the development of insulin-resistance. Insulin-resistance is a condition in which the body is unable to use insulin effectively to regulate blood sugar. This is a primary factor in diabetes. Stress can also exacerbate existing diabetes levels by impairing the patient's ability to manage the disease effectively with dietary restrictions, exercise and other lifestyle changes.

Pain

The perception of pain is exaggerated by stress. Researchers have established a relationship between pain and emotion. It is well known that chronic pain caused by arthritis and other degenerative disorders is intensified by stress. Stress also plays a significant role in the severity of back pain. Backache and neck pain are often a result of faulty postures created by stress. There is also a strong association between depression and back problems. Headaches such as tension headaches and migraines often have their genesis in some form of stress. A constant frown created by stress can lead to tension headaches.

Sexual Dysfunction
Stress can cause erectile dysfunction in men. This is caused by lack of desire due to tension or due to problem with the blood flow to the penis. The stress hormones constrict the arteries to the penis causing reduced blood flow needed for erection. The stress response also increases the blood flow out of the penis which can prevent erection. Stress can lead to diminished sexual desire and an inability to achieve orgasm in women.

Infertility and Menstrual Problems
Stress may even affect fertility. Stress has an impact on the hypothalamus, which indirectly regulates the production of reproductive hormones. In extreme conditions, severely elevated cortisol levels can even shut down menstruation. One interesting study reported a significantly higher incidence of infertility in women who experienced both high stress and prolonged menstrual cycles.

Stress and Pregnancy
Stress during pregnancy has been linked to a higher risk for miscarriage, lower birth weights, and increased incidence of premature births. Indeed, one study found a higher rate of crying and low attention span in infants of mothers who had been stressed during pregnancy.

Skin Disorders
Stress has been related to a host of skin conditions. Skin allergies, acne, psoriasis, eczema etc are precipitated due to stress. In fact skin allergies are caused more by stress than due to pollutants and other external factors.

CHAPTER 4 : ILL EFFECTS OF STRESS

Hair Fall

Stress has been held responsible for a condition called Alopecia Areata. In this condition there is hair loss that occurs in localized patches. Stress is also associated with generalized hair loss or balding. Hair loss often occurs during periods of intense stress, such as during the period of mourning or any other kind of loss and setback.

Teeth and Gums

Studies show that stress and periodontal disease are connected. Stress has now been implicated in increasing the risk for periodontal disease where the gums are affected adversely. The disease may progress to cause a loss of teeth.

EFFECTS OF STRESS ON BEHAVIOURAL PATTERNS

Alcoholism

Alcohol affects receptors in the brain that reduce stress. This is the reason people under chronic stress frequently seek relief through alcohol abuse. The calming effects of alcohol are temporary and the stressed person is worse off after the effect of alcohol has passed. Over time, tolerance is developed towards alcohol, where more quantities are needed to soothe the nerves. This can lead to dependence and alcoholism.

Smoking

Stress causes excessive smoking. Often taken under peer pressure or under the effect of popular media stereotypes, the nicotine habit is hard to shake off and often shoots up during stress. There are studies that have indicated that nicotine has a calming effect in humans. Deprivation of nicotine increases stress in smokers, which creates a cycle of dependency. Smoking, in turn, can cause a plethora of health problems ranging from heart attacks to lung cancer.

Concentration and Memory

Some amount of optimal stress has been shown to be beneficial for achieving concentration. This is the BP zone or the **Zone of Best**

Performance. Prolonged stress, however, affects the ability to concentrate and perform. Attention deficit syndrome caused by stress is well known. School children who are stressed are shown to have short attention spans leading to poor grades in studies. Stress affects memory adversely. Both short term and long term memory suffer at the hands of stress.

Eating Problems
Obesity as well as excessive weight loss can be brought about by stress. Anorexia nervosa and bulimia have a strong connection with stress. These conditions have been known to respond to stress management programmes like relaxation, deep breathing and meditation.

Weight gain and obesity can be linked to stress. Tension creates craving for the wrong kinds of food. People who are stressed resort to sweets, fat and junk food laden with salt and put on weight. Weight gain can occur even with a healthy diet, in some people exposed to stress. This weight precipitated by the stress hormones usually accumulates in the abdominal area.

Sleep Disturbances
Stress can alter sleep patterns. The quantity and quality of sleep often suffer due to stress. Stress can cause insomnia where the stressed person is kept awake till late hours. Stress can also cause awakening in the middle of the night or in the early hours of the morning with poor success in getting back to sleep.

> The stress response, which starts in the mind, ultimately goes on to involve the whole body. The stressed brain starts a cascade of hormonal activity, which has damaging consequences to our health.

Can Stress be Helpful?

CHAPTER 5

Adopting the right attitude can convert a negative stress into a positive one — Hans Selye

John McEnroe, the former tennis star, thrived under pressure. In fact, a tight situation often brought out the best in him. It can be rightly said, in his case, that he romanced stress. Sample this...an important match like the Wimbledon Final...John McEnroe... leveled scores and a bad line call... this would be the perfect setting for the famous McEnroe outburst! While the world would be at the edge of their seats, John McEnroe, tennis's very own, original bad boy would work himself up. His temper would fly, swear words would be hurtled and the racket would be flung. Pumping himself into a frenzy, he would fire the best serve of the match. This is an example of how stress may actually bring out the best in an individual. Such stress is called Eustress.

Stress need not always emanate from negative instances. A positive event such as a promotion at work, a move to a new neighbourhood or marriage in the family can also produce reactions that are stressful. However, since the events or the stressors are positive, so also their aftermath. Such stressors bring in a lot of enjoyment and satisfaction and build up a zest for life. This variety of positive stress has been labelled as **Eustress** to distinguish it from negative stress, or **Distress**.

> The nervous excitement encountered on your first date is Eustress and what follows is Distress.
> *Baba Calm Dev*

I too have experienced eustress or good stress many times. I have felt it as butterflies in the stomach before a music concert, before starting a surgery using a new technique and also before putting on the 18th green. This good stress motivated, energized and, most often than not, increased the level and quality of performance.

Good stress is as much a reality as bad stress. One gives you energy and passion; the other wrecks your health and robs you of your vitality and zest for life. Trying to make a positive out of a negative event is the real challenge before us individuals. The stress-related state of physiological arousal can actually improve concentration, performance and efficiency. Some people actually do their best work when they are under pressure. They relax when they have met the challenge, take pride in their accomplishment, and gear up for the next project. Thus, they view 'achievement under pressure' as a kind of positive stress that is satisfying and rewarding. Another example is where deadlines are used to motivate people who seem bored or demotivated. Once the deadline is fixed, the student or the worker gears up for the event and goes full throttle.

So long as stress is within our control, it has benefits. The same stress when it assumes greater magnitude, remains persistent and starts affecting the mental and physical health of a person, it is then considered to be damaging. As long as our self-analysis yields that the situation is in our control, stress is perceived as eustress. It can be used by individuals to power themselves and gain more control over situations in their life. However, what is eustress and what is not often depends on the person's self-analysis and assessment of the resources he has in hand. A wrong assessment may lead to a failure thereby, setting off a chain of events that may be hugely non-conducive to individual health and zest for life.

THE BEST PERFORMANCE ZONE

The relationship between stress and performance is explained by the graph. Performance forms the vertical axis and pressure forms the horizontal axis. The Inverted-U figure defines the relationship between pressure and performance and signifies the change in level of performance as the pressure rises.

The left half of the graph shows the positive effect of stress on performance. When there is very little pressure or stress, there is hardly any motivation to perform. As the stress level increases, our ability to perform too begins to pick up. As pressure on us increases further, we enter the **Best Performance Zone**. At this stage we are able to completely focus on the task with a vigour that produces great results. At this level there is enough pressure to stimulate us but not so much that it disrupts our performance. The right half of the graph with a downward slope signifies that when the pressure mounts and persists beyond the critical limit of an individual, the performance plummets.

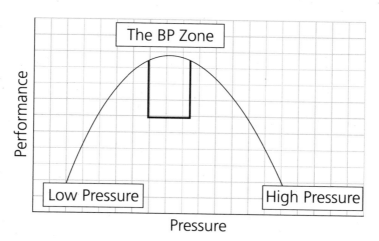

HOW DOES ONE USE EUSTRESS TO BEST ADVANTAGE?

Since it is difficult to eliminate stress, one can learn to manage it. You should be able to determine the level of stress that is optimal for you. The key is to find a moderate level of arousal that works for you so as to achieve a state of eustress. Arousal is the energy eustress provides us. However if you're too aroused, you're likely to get into distress and fall apart. On the other hand, if you're not aroused enough, you won't be in eustress and won't be able to get much done.

So what constitutes the right amount of stress? There is no definite answer to this. It is very individualistic and depends on your personality, the amount of stress you can endure, and the task at hand. As a surgeon or a golfer, I need to sustain lower stress levels. Higher levels would induce muscle tightness and tremor, and that will affect the action. On the other hand, if I need to sing or perform in front of a large audience I need to rev up the energy levels to get the best from my stage performance and reach out to the person in the last row.

The key, therefore, is to identify the productive stress zone or the best performance zone for yourself, especially in light of the activity you are to perform. Your presence in this zone will ensure the right dose of motivation and help you attain success. In addition, it will keep the negative effects of stress at bay.

> Some stress is needed to rev up our performance, but too much is disastrous. If we learn to identify this optimum level of stress, we will be in the desired Zone of Best Performance.

CHAPTER 6

The Calm Sutra
Stress Busters

I think we have spent enough time discussing stress and its effects, both positive and negative. The positive effects of stress are not the ones that need intervention; those that need some amount of looking into are the negative effects emanating from stress and it is about time we did something about it.

As stated earlier, stress management can be achieved through a combination of processes; building awareness, adopting a proactive attitude; accepting life; learning to live in the moment and taking action by opting for stress-busting techniques.

Through the process of thought awareness and proactive attitude we can try to identify the stressors. We can plan things in advance, set realistic goals and avoid situations which are potential stressors. I have tried to deal with proactive attitude in another chapter.

Just as we saw that stress can bring about changes in the body, similarly bodily actions can bring about a favourable reduction in the stress levels. Just as there are psycho-somatic disorders, so also there are somato-psychic manoeuvers or actions, which can come in handy while managing stress. These manoeuvers include breathing techniques, postural disciplines, visualization and affirmation routines and many other enjoyable activities. It also includes physical

> You can fish best when the boat is steady.
> *Baba Calm Dev*

exercises. As stated earlier, all these techniques are therapeutic and help in bringing down stress levels and preserve the strength and vitality of the physical self.

Many a times it is not possible to completely eliminate stressors or unfavourable situations in life. However, with some strategies one can lessen the impact of stress. Most of these techniques keep us rooted to the present and in this they preserve a sense of continuity and thwart disjointedness in the mind and body connection.

While discussing stress and mind-body connection, we saw that our body produced stress hormones which had disastrous effects on our body. The body becomes prey to a plethora of illnesses and is unable to repair without minus interventions.

Stress reduction or defense building techniques, as we will call them, release another group of chemicals or molecules that heal and, bring a calming effect on the body and mind. These are called **endorphins** and are produced when we exercise, meditate or have sex. These are elixirs that work like magic and bring about intrinsic upliftment, peace and happiness. Endorphins are responsible for the feeling of being 'high' or on 'top of the world'. Take for example, an athlete who completes a tough race. The happiness experienced by the runner is compared to an orgasm. He enters a higher state of happiness. This is the handiwork of the endorphins that are released. Persons indulging in chanting or meditation also experience a similar phenomenon. Again, it is the endorphins that are responsible for people going in a trance during a tribal dance, where it is difficult to tell the dancer from the dance. Most of the stress busters have some kind of an endorphin effect, which makes them effective and almost addictive.

Most stress busters described here are successful because they serve the purpose they are made for, that is they aid in reducing stress. In addition, they engage a person's mind and thereby, leave very little scope for worry or tension.

COMMON STRESS BUSTERS

Some of the more common aids used by people to deal with stress are given below. This is not an exhaustive list, rather a compilation of some of the more common stress busting techniques that people use.

Body-Mind Exercises
- Deep breathing
- Progressive muscle relaxation
- Stretching
- Yoga
- Aerobics
- Weight training
- Mind games like the sudoku, chess, crosswords, puzzles, vedic mathematics
- Sex
- Posture training

Sports: All Kinds of Sports, but usually
- Golf
- Tennis
- Table Tennis
- Badminton
- Swimming

Hobbies and Art Forms
- Music
- Dance
- Painting
- Gardening

Mind Drills
- Meditation
- Visualization
- Affirmations
- Hypnosis

Dietary Habits
- Meditative eating
- Balanced eating
- Good hydration

Life enriching Measures
- Vacationing
- Forming meaningful relationships
- Resorting to humour
- Going to the spa, or to a masseur

The list is certainly not exhaustive and individuals may find certain other tasks more apt and therapeutic in accordance to their needs.

WHY SO MANY STRESS BUSTERS?

There is an old dictum in surgery, 'If there are too many techniques to do an operation possibly none of them works'.

However, I do not think that the same holds true for these anti stress measures. Too many stress busting measures are actually good for the individual as he has an array to choose from. What he finally opts for depends on his personality, body type, needs, attitudes, and state of the mind, interest, energy levels, cultural background and the likes.

Some of the techniques like meditation, hypnosis, creative visualization need far more intensive efforts and a more concentrated frame of mind to be effective, whereas activities like walking and laughing can be done by almost everybody and needs less of concentrated efforts.

Again, activities like golf and tennis need both, the physical facilities and the finance, but visualization and imagery can be done while sitting in your drawing room.

Yoga, dance and progressive muscle relaxation need training whereas chilling out with good friends, having a fun time just requires you to take some time out for them.

CHAPTER 6 : THE CALM SUTRA STRESS BUSTERS

As long as you have the resource and the inclination you can choose one or more of the techniques listed above to make life more relaxed and stress free. You can also go a step ahead and invent your own method of relaxation.

I have seen two very diverse methods of stress management in my parents. My mother is very religious, meditates and tries to remain in the moment. Her ability to enjoy every moment has led her to try various activities from high-level table tennis to candle making to magic.

On the other hand, my father who is a confirmed atheist, has no inclination towards religion and spiritualism. He has a typical type B personality, which somehow does not attract stressors. He is the one with proactive attitude to life. "If you cannot stop the noise, wear ear plugs", is his attitude.

The stress management formula, my parents have had in common, has been involvement in sporting activity.

HAVE YOU TAKEN THE INJECTION DOC?

A couple of years ago I was performing a knee ligament reconstruction surgery at Lilavati Hospital, Mumbai. The patient was a young Englishman who had injured his knee while indulging in water sports in Goa. He was a cheerful young man, till he entered the operation theatre. Once on the operation table he looked pale and petrified. I explained the surgical steps to him, the rehabilitation programme etc, which he understood quite well. When it came to explaining the anaesthesia technique, I told him that he would be getting a tiny needle prick in his back, which would make his legs go numb. To pacify him, I told him that the injection was not a big deal and absolutely painless.

At this juncture he erupted and asked me, "Have you taken the injection doc?"

I said "No, but..."

"With due respect to you doc, if you have not taken the injection, you have no idea what it is. I have taken it twice before and know how painful it is."

His reply had me dumbfounded for a minute. There was no fight or flight situation here. Rather it was a just-face-it-and-finish-it kind of a situation.

Why am I telling you all this? Well, all the techniques of stress management that I have described in this book, I have tried them out. All of these are tested ways to beat stress. Yes, this time, I have taken the injection...

> Stress busters include a huge number of activities like meditation, deep breathing, music, dance, sex, exercise, chilling out with friends, and of course golf. Take your pick and have a ball.

CHAPTER 7

Proactive Attitude

God grant us the serenity to accept the things we cannot change, courage to change the things we can, and wisdom to know the difference — Dr. Rheinhold Niebuhr

Proactivity is one of the most popular management buzzwords that has come up in the 1990s. The credit for popularizing proactivity or proactive behaviour should go to Stephen Covey.

Though commonly used, there are a number of definitions for the term 'Proactivity'. Different people have interpreted the term differently. For many, the term proactive would mean taking action on an issue before being asked. So actually, proactive people are individuals who take initiatives and often assume leadership roles.

Stephen Covey, in his best selling book *The 7 Habits of Highly Effective People* urges readers to 'be proactive'. Proactivity heads the list of seven habits which are guaranteed to make you successful and happy. He defines proactivity as more than merely taking the initiative; instead he focuses on **response-ability** - the ability and freedom to choose a response in reaction to a stimulus.

> Unavoidable exertion is bonus exercise.
> *Baba Calm Dev*

THE CALM PAUSE CONCEPT

To understand proactivity one must first know what reactivity is. Reactive behaviour comes from providing an immediate, impulsive and many times thoughtless reflex reaction to stimulation. In proactive behaviour there is a pause between stimulus and response. The pause is used for making a suitable choice of response.

For example, a poisonous snake bites a person. If the person is reactive, his reaction would be to kill the snake. However, if he is proactive, he will not be impulsive, rather he will give some thought to the situation at hand and take recourse to a medical centre for treatment. Both individuals are scared, hurt and in pain. What sets the two apart is that the proactive person takes a pause, a calm pause. This pause gives him enough time and opportunity to make a correct decision, sometimes (as in this case) a life saving decision.

Proactive behaviour can save many situations and avoid a lot of unpleasantness. For example, in the operation theatre things can often go wrong. During a key step in surgery, a nurse drops a vital instrument. In a reactive reaction, the surgeon loses his temper, shouts at the nurse and there is chaos. The nurse gets more nervous and is capable of dropping more instruments.

A proactive surgeon, on the other hand, takes a calm pause, and asks everybody to relax. He then asks the scrub nurse for a replacement for the dropped instrument and carries on with the surgery.

At the end of the surgery, the protocol of passing instruments correctly is discussed, and necessary steps are taken to ensure that the event is not repeated. Proactive attitude not only reduces stress in a person, but also in those around him. In fact, a proactive leader can change the entire social fabric.

Lack of proactivity often leads to road rage, which is a typical example of reactive behaviour.

On the topic of road rage, I want to share with you a phenomenon called autorickshaw or rickshaw, fondly called rik by some. In some other South Asian countries it is referred to as a "tuk-tuk", a name derived from the sound it produces. It is a three wheeler and a good mode of public transport for the middle class.

It is the driver of the rik who fascinates me. He believes he is Michael Schumacher and Valentino Rossi rolled into one with powers

CHAPTER 7 : PROACTIVE ATTITUDE

of Batman and Lord Hanuman put together. He has scant respect for signal lights, pedestrian crossings, road dividers, no parking zones or any other traffic regulation you can think of. He uses his dexterity to weave between cars, takes amazing U-turns in the minimum of space, he brakes at a split second notice, changing lanes is child's play for him and so is driving on the wrong side of the road. When he is being good he is driving at 20 kmph in the outer lane!

Now, when one of these "riks" suddenly swerves in your path the typical reaction is:

How dare he cut me? I will teach the ba....d a lesson. These rickshaws should be wiped off the streets, let me begin with this one. And the rage begins, which often ends with dire consequences. What is needed here is a "Calm Pause", which is usually accompanied by a deep breath. The pause gives you a chance to provide a proactive response. The proactive person would first get out of harms way and then think further. Very often no further action is needed.

THE HUMOUR OPTION

Proactive attitude can go a step further and view the situation with a touch of humour, as does Baba Calm Dev. Baba in a lighter vein has suggested a fantastic "sci-fi" script to Hollywood where one mutant autorickshaw finds its way into America. Like some pesky protozoan it splits itself and starts multiplying. Soon you have millions of riks on super ways, turnpikes, and downtown avenues. They invade the White House, the Capitol and the senate to create chaos of a different kind!

PROACTIVE AFFIRMATIONS

I was lucky to have been on the faculty for a youth leadership programme organized by the Forum of Free Enterprise in Mumbai. At this programme proactive responses were discussed with practical applications. At this programme it was concluded that a proactive person or leader should make the following affirmations and believe in them.

I am Calm.
There are abundant opportunities that await me.
I feel in charge to make things happen.
I feel responsible for my own life.
I take the initiative.
I am able to choose my own actions.

THINGS I CAN CHANGE

Apart from choosing the appropriate response to a stimulus, a proactive person focuses on things under his control. This concept has been beautifully explained by Stephen Covey in his book, *The 7 Habits of Highly Effective People*. He has emphasized on the circle of concern and the circle of influence as a way to attain proactive attitude.

The circle of concern deals with the problems at hand, or the sources of worry i.e. stressors. The circle of influence deals with the power we possess to alter the circle of concern. If our circle of influence overshadows the circle of concern, we are proactive and happy. If the circle of concern dominates our life, we are usually under stress.

LET US TRY AND UNDERSTAND THIS BEAUTIFUL CONCEPT.

First Scenario:

There is noise in the neighbourhood. Stray dogs keep barking at night and I am not able to sleep. This is a concern, a worry.

Can I change this situation?

Yes, the circle of influence suggests that I complain to the local authorities and have the dogs removed. I can change this situation; it is in my circle of influence.

Second Scenario:

There is noise at night and it is caused by airplanes flying over my house. The options are to write to the Ministry for Aviation and have the planes rerouted or simply wear ear plugs. The path of the

CHAPTER 7 : PROACTIVE ATTITUDE

planes cannot be changed. This has to be accepted. What is in my control though is to reduce the noise at my end.

As Dr. Covey states that proactive people focus their efforts within their circle of influence. They work on the things that they can initiate changes in. The nature of their energy is positive, enlarging and magnifying, causing their circle of influence to constantly increase.

Reactive people, on the other hand, focus their efforts in the circle of concern or on the things they cannot change. They focus on the weakness of other people, the problems in the environment, and circumstances over which they have no control. Their focus results in blaming and accusing others, using abusive language, and increased feelings of victimization. This negative energy brings on a vicious circle and causes their circle of influence to shrink.

BEST OUT ADVERSITY

Going a step further proactive people can reap benefit, even from an adverse situation. I remember when we were medical students we had gone to Goa for an inter-medical cultural festival. After our act was over, some of us got so involved in accepting accolades, that we missed the last bus to our accommodation. We had to walk back about 6 kilometers at night. Though the concept of proactive and reactive attitude was not known then, I can look back and identify the two groups by the response. The reactive ones among us started cursing the ones responsible for the delay. The stupid organization, the pathetic bus system in Goa, and whatever else they could think of. Crib, walk, crib trudge, crib drag... was what they did.

The proactive ones however enjoyed the cool night and the long walk. For me, even today, it is beautiful trip down memory lane. Whenever Rashmi, my wife, and I visit Goa we identify the spot, from where we began that romantic and bonding walk together.

THE 'WORST CASE SCENARIO' CONCEPT

When something is evidently going wrong, worrying about it does not help. In fact, worry reduces our ability to concentrate on the task at hand, causing the situation to get worse. Worry begets a haphazard thought process and we lose the ability to make good decisions. We can only improve a bad situation if we can focus all of our attention on the task.

I remember, a tense table-tennis match during my medical college days. The rivalry between medical colleges in Mumbai was not limited to academics. The rivalry bordering on enemity often spilt onto the sports arena. I was playing against a relatively unknown player from a rival medical college. I was the ranked player and was under pressure to wrap the match easily. However, the crowds from the opponent's college out-numbered ours and amidst the booing and heckling, I soon found myself trailing the match badly. The embarrasment of being beaten by a novice in enemy territory put more pressure on me and I choked badly. I succumbed to the stress and ended up losing the match. I am sure if I had acted proactively and accepted the fact that losing the match was not the end of the world, I could have concentrated on the task on hand and fared better.

Here are some steps we can take to accept the worst case scenario and work it in our favour.

Envisage the Worst-Case Scenario
Realizing the worst possible outcome will help put things in perspective and come to terms with an adverse situation. Stuck in traffic, the worst case scenario is that you will be late to work. Nothing more. Putting on the 18th green, worst case scenario, you might miss the putt. Nothing more.

It is Not the End of the World, Accept It
Once you have determined the worst-case scenario, you need to mentally accept it. Assume that it is going to happen. So what if it happens, it is not the end of the world. You are not going to die or be put behind bars in any case. If you are resigned to the fact that the worst outcome is not the end of the world, then you can stop worrying. There is an immediate release of stress when you accept

the worst case scenario. After you accept the situation, you can move on to the next step.

Improve the Worst-Case Scenario
Now that you are free from worrying about the outcome, you can devote your full attention towards improving it. Try to find ways to reduce the negative effects of the outcome. You may not be able to turn a losing situation into a winning situation, but you might be able to make it neutral or at the very least, less bad.

PRACTICAL PROACTIVITY
Thus in summation, we can state that walking the path of proactivity is not at all difficult. In fact, it can be done by following some simple steps like taking a calm pause, accepting the situation, focusing on the things you can change and deliberating on those you cannot, adopting a positive frame of mind; all of these aid in furthering the path of practical proactivity.

> Six ways to walk the path of Practical Proactivity:
> - Take a calm pause
> - Look for the humour option
> - Make positive affirmations
> - Focus on things you can change
> - Make the best out of adversity
> - Work on the worst case scenario

CALM SUTRA : THE ART OF RELAXATION

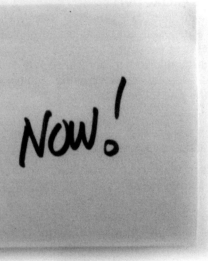

Being in the Present

CHAPTER 8

Forget about your life situation and pay attention to your life. Your life situation exists in time. Your life is now. — Eckhart Tolle in his book, *The Power of Now*.

This book is very enlightening and encourages people to live in the present. For us Indians this is not an altogether alien concept. Gautam Buddha is known to have said, "Do not dwell in the past; do not dream of the future, concentrate the mind on the present moment." Clearly, the concept of 'now' is an important one.

Our mind is really a 'one track mind'. Unlike music editing machines where several tracks play at one time, our mind can have one thought or a feeling at one time. The music editing machine can play the strings on one track, drums on another, guitar on the third and many such instruments simultaneously, to make great music. The mind, however, cannot do two things at the same time. You can either enjoy the succulence of the tandoori chicken or you can catch the punch line in 'Friends', the sitcom. If your mind is registering the succulence to the fullest, the punch line is gone. You turn to your wife and ask her "what happened?" As she turns to explain what happened, the next punch line is gone! If you are immersed in the punch lines the succulence of your tandoori chicken is lost. Then it boils down to a great show on TV and some tandoori chicken. The enjoyment one

> Make your present felt, to yourself.
> *Baba Calm Dev*

CALM SUTRA : THE ART OF RELAXATION

could have had from doing things separately is gone.

"To enjoy life to the fullest one needs to be right in the present. Now. Here. Or else we would be nowhere." says Baba Calm Dev.

Not many years ago when Rashmi, my wife, and I were 18 and dating, we would go to eat some fabulous sizzlers every month. We would save from our pocket money and make the trip to a South Bombay sizzler joint. The food was superb and the atmosphere was divine. The only complaint Rashmi had was that I would pay very little attention to her. I would be totally immersed in the sizzler and hardly look up. In retrospect, maybe I was living life in those moments. The power of the moment had me in its grip.

Being in the present moment can bring out the best in an individual. It forces him to be totally involved and the work at hand greatly benefits from this kind of involvement.

In the operation theatre we play soft music. This soothes the patients and works towards smooth induction of anesthesia. As soon as the patient is under anesthesia and surgery is to start, I request for the music to be put off. That is because, being passionate about music, I find it difficult to concentrate and a surgical procedure does need all the attention I can muster. So I am better off without the music in my operation theatre. However, music is a great accompaniment while I am driving or dancing or exercising or simply lounging.

As you learn to live in the moment, you will start enjoying life more. You will find yourself more attentive, innovative and creative and perform better at any given task. A lot of negativity will disappear. Most activities will then become easier and less stressful, perhaps also fun when you decide to live your life in its moments and not fret over what is to come or what has gone by. Only then will happiness be up for grabs.

LOSING THE MOMENT

Losing the moment is very common. It happens to all of us, at some point in our lives or another. Whether it is while watching a movie or while attending a lecture, our minds tend to wander and we lose

CHAPTER 8 : BEING IN THE PRESENT

connection with what is happening. The mind usually hooks on to a word or an event and goes into the past. The word or the event takes our thought to a similar event in our experience and what follows is chain or a cascade of thoughts. This leads to a phenomenon called Mental Chatter or Brownian Movement of Thoughts. This chatter takes us away, from the present, into a different time and space zone. Not only do we lose precious information, but the gaps in information leave us stressed too.

When we come back to the moment due to some interruption or due to our own awareness, we get the feeling, "Hey where was I? I have missed something."

RETURNING TO THE MOMENT: AA OF CALM SUTRA

Being in the moment is possible with the help of the skills: Awareness and Action.

Awareness of our self and our thought process can bring us back in the moment. Awareness is a skill one can develop with a certain amount of practice. If we develop awareness of our bodies we can notice if we are sitting, standing or carrying weights correctly. If we develop awareness of our breathing, we can notice whether our breathing is deep or shallow. Similarly if we develop awareness of our thoughts, we will know whether we are in the moment or not and get our thoughts organized.

Once this awareness is generated, we can begin to prioritize and streamline our actions. Being aware of our thoughts is called Sakshi Bhaav in the *Bhagvad Gita*. If we develop the ability to watch our thoughts and our actions, our chances of proactivity increases.

After awareness comes **Action**. Once aware, a person can take remedial action if necessary. For example if we are aware that our posture is not correct, we take remedial steps in this direction. The same is true with breathing and thinking. Once we have the ability of being aware of our thoughts we can gently guide them to the present. We can bring the thoughts back to the moment instead of letting them wander. We can even learn to monitor our responses to a particular stimulus and avoid an unfavorable reaction.

REMINISCING AND DREAMING BEING IN THE MOMENT

Does it mean that by being in the moment, I am not allowed to make plans for the future or reflect on the past? Could I be in the moment and yet be thinking about the past or the future?

The answer to both these questions is 'yes' since the idea is to live in the moment, not be stuck to the moment.

Actually, being in the moment means being mindfully aware of what is going on right here and now. There are ways of mindfully thinking about the past or future. We can mindfully and creatively call to mind past events and savour all the good memories. It is fantastic to go back and recollect all the stories my great grand mother told me or the musical variations sung by my aunt. There are beautiful memories, which can be reconstructed and relived. Many of these memories can be brought to life with their associated sounds, fragrances and textures. If a certain song is played, my thoughts go back in time when it was popular, especially to events around that time. I can see the people of that time, the fragrant food being prepared, my school bag being packed. All this is seen and felt, in the magnificent theatre of my mind.

What should be avoided, however, is brooding over the past. We tend to get lost in our thoughts and are confused. This line of thinking can create a lot of stress. When we think about the future, it should be done with a purpose else it tends to become idle day dreaming. Setting goals is a purposeful activity and it helps sets goals for us.

Most of the meditative techniques and other Stress Busters described in Calm Sutra help us remain in the moment.

> Life can be enjoyed abundantly, by being in the moment. Being in the moment allows us no time to brood over the past or fear the unknown of the future. Enjoy the gift, the Present, NOW.

Deep Breathing

CHAPTER 9

Breathing and life go hand in hand. One cannot exist without the other. Breath in Sanskrit is Praana, which denotes life. Breathing, like the beating of the heart, starts with birth and goes on till the day one dies. Breathing just goes on and on without stopping. However, unlike the heart beat, over which we have no direct control, breathing can be controlled by us, so as to add more vitality to our health and lives.

Our bodies cannot do without air, essentially oxygen and this is why breathing assumes paramount importance. Air is nourishment to our bodies just as much as food and water is. Air gives our blood the supply of oxygen it must have in order to feed itself. That, in turn, feed the tissues, nerves, glands and vital organs. Without oxygen even our skin, bones, teeth and hair would not remain properly conditioned. Our digestion also fails without oxygen. However, most importantly, our mental faculties slow down, feel sluggish and finally fail in the absence of oxygen.

Inhalation as well as exhalation is important and the human body is designed to discharge 70% of its toxins through the process of exhalation. Only a small percentage of toxins are discharged through sweat, defecation and urination. If your breathing is not operating at peak efficiency, you are not ridding yourself of toxins properly which is really harmful to the body.

> Some *Breathtaking* information in store for you.
> *Baba Calm Dev*

In a single day we breathe about 23,000 times at an approximate average of 16 breaths a minute. The average volumes of air taken in with a single breath is about 20 cubic inches, depending on a person's size, sex, posture, the nature of the surrounding atmosphere and one's physical and emotional state. However, with proper attention given to breathing, this volume may be increased to 100 or even 130 cubic inches per breath. With proper breathing exercises and techniques you can provide yourself 5 times more oxygen and get rid of 5 times the carbon dioxide you would normally exhale.

THE BASIC BREATHING MECHANISM

Proper breathing is performed with the mouth closed so that the air is inhaled through your nose. The air travels down the pharynx or the throat, the larynx or the voice box and the trachea or windpipe until it reaches the air sacs or alveoli via the bronchial tubes.

The breathing mechanism works through the nose and follows certain essential steps. Firstly, the dust and bacteria are filtered out by the hair and moist mucus membrane, which lines the nasal passage. The mucus membrane in the nose, apart from filtering substances, also has certain germicidal properties. When we breathe through our nose, the passage to the lungs is longer than we breathe through our mouth. While traveling through this longer passage the air is warmed up to a proper body temperature.

After being filtered and warmed thus, the supply of air moves on from the bronchi straight into the lungs. Here it enters millions of cells called alveoli, which are tiny air sacs. Surrounding these sacs is a network of equally tiny blood vessels or capillaries. The blood absorbs the fresh oxygen directly through the cell walls just as it rids of the carbon-di-oxide.

Next the freshly oxygenated blood or the pure blood, travels to the heart. The heart pumps the blood via arteries to every part of the body supplying oxygen and nutrition to every organ and every tissue to the last bone cell. A huge amount of blood passes through the heart and lungs every hour. So the heart and the lungs are put

CHAPTER 9 : DEEP BREATHING

to a lot of hard work during the entire span of one's life.

POOR BREATHING HABITS

"Insufficient oxygen means insufficient biological energy that can result in anything from mild fatigue to life-threatening disease." ~ W. Spencer Way, Journal of the American Association of Physicians

As babies we breathe deeply, laugh heartily and cry out passionately. As we grow up we start developing bad habits. We breathe shallow, laugh rarely and are too shy to cry. The more educated and experienced we get, we lose some of the good habits we had as children. We think too much, worry unnecessarily, slouch, eat even when we are not hungry and do many more things wrongly.

Although we all breathe, few of us retain the habit of full breathing referred to as Diaphragmatic Breathing. As the average person reaches middle age, lung tissues tend to grow less and less elastic. Years of habitual thoracic breathing can take its toll on the chest wall, which loses its flexibility and becomes rigid. The sequel to this is an accumulation of waste products in the blood stream, which often leads to those vague syndromes of pain and discomfort. These symptoms are often considered vague and busy doctors have little time to treat these. Many of the backaches and headaches fall into this category. Hence proper breathing is a must for the maintenance of the body and its regulation.

STRESS AND BREATHING

Most of us unconsciously breathe from our chest or thorax. However, during stress, it is the thoracic breathing that comes into play. Thoracic breathing supplies insufficient oxygen to the blood, which causes the heart and lungs to work harder to accomplish the proper amount of oxygenation. Thoracic breathers will require 16 - 20 breaths per minute while diaphragmatic breathers require only 6 - 8 breaths per minute. Hence it is not very conducive to one's health. In fact, the workload on the heart and lungs can be reduced by half, when we switch from thoracic to diaphragmatic breathing. Thus diaphragmatic breathing increases the efficiency of the entire cardio-respiratory functioning.

During stress there are two types of breathing that is produced. In acute stress the breathing becomes rapid, shallow and could cause hyperventilation. In chronic stress, there is inhibited breathing where the rate as well as the depth fall. This leads to chronic hypoventilation and all other associated health problems.

BUILDING BREATH AWARENESS

Breath awareness teaches us to pay attention to our breathing habits. To improve the breathing pattern it is essential to first be aware of our breathing habits.

Begin with switching off your cell phone. Sit comfortably but erect, with a back rest. The following points are to be noted:

1) Posture: One of the most important aspects, which contribute to bad breathing, is bad posture. If we are slouched, with hunched shoulders and crouched spine, the diaphragm does not get a chance to complete its excursion. The lungs do not get to expand completely, nor do they achieve complete exhalation. A relaxed posture with the buttocks touching the backrest of the chair, shoulders square and back straight, is desirable.

2) Deep and Abdominal: Analyse your breath. Is the breath shallow or deep, is it long or short? The best way to find out whether it is abdominal or thoracic is by keeping a hand on the chest and the other on the tummy. While taking a deep breath the hand on the tummy must rise with each inhalation and fall with each exhalation.

3) Slow or Fast: The rate of respiration is determined by counting the number of breaths per minute. The average number of breaths in an adult is around 16 breaths a minute. Persons who are deep diaphragmatic breathers could have a rate of around 6 breaths a minute.

4) Pauses: There are two distinct pauses, one between inhalation and exhalation and another between exhalation and inhalation. These are natural pauses even when there is no breath holding.

5) The Ratio of Inhalation to Exhalation: The time taken for

CHAPTER 9 : DEEP BREATHING

breathing in and the time taken for breathing out can be monitored. Are they of equal duration or is the exhalation longer than the inhalation. Awareness of breath must include such points.

6) Are you Breathing from the Nose or Mouth: There are habitual nose breathers and habitual mouth breathers. Awareness in the breathing method will tell us whether we are breathing correctly through our nose or not.

All this will make us aware of our breathing style and help us rectify things, if required. Breathing properly is very important, probably as important as breathing itself. Hence a precise analysis is a pre-requisite to proper intervention. This can bring down stress levels and aid in a healthier individual.

BASIC BREATHING EXERCISE

Breath plays a prominent role in whether or not we suffer from stress. Proper breathing is an antidote to stress. Apart from improving your breathing, this exercise will help you become more aware of your breathing process.

Step One

Improve your Posture: Sit in a comfortable position, have a backrest, but keep your back straight. Select a place, where you are not likely to be disturbed. Loose clothing is preferred.

Place your right hand on your abdomen, with the little finger just above your navel.

Place your left hand on your upper chest with the little finger between your breasts.

Step Two

Become Conscious/Aware: Become aware of your breathing as you inhale and exhale. Feel the air enter through your nostrils and pass your throat into the chest. Concentrate on the air moving down into your abdomen as if you were filling your belly with air. Mind you this is an illusion that the air is going into your abdomen. As long as you are not swallowing the air, it enters your lungs. The abdomen moves to facilitate the movement of the diaphragm so that the lungs can expand fully.

Step Three
Ensure that the Breath is Deep and Abdominal: As you breathe in, your right hand should rise. As you exhale, your right hand should fall. Your left hand should be moving very little. Within a few moments, you will become more comfortable with this type of breathing. Do not try to force the breath. Allow the motion to be effortless and gentle. Pay close attention to the ease with which you breathe deeply, easily, and smoothly.

This is diaphragmatic breathing. Now, as you continue practising diaphragmatic breathing, I want you to concentrate on making the breath smooth and even. The inhalation and exhalation should be of the same length and pressure. Try not to exhale all of the air out at the start of exhalation. Allow it to flow evenly throughout the cycle. Relax and allow irregularities, in your breathing to fade away as your breathing becomes easy, even, and smooth. Imagine the breath is like a wheel moving without any jerks. Evenly and smoothly.

Step Four
Prolong Exhalation: Now that you are feeling relaxed and your breathing is slow and rhythmic, gently slow down the rate of exhalation so that you are breathing out twice as long as you are breathing in. Do not try to fill your lungs completely, or empty them completely.

You simply want to alter the rhythm of the breathing.

You may try counting to 8 as you exhale, and 4 as you inhale.

After you have established the new rhythm, stop the mental counting and focus again on the smoothness and evenness of your breath. Continue to breathe this way for the next five minutes focusing on the smooth, even rhythm of your breathing.

CHAPTER 9 : DEEP BREATHING

MORE BREATHING EXERCISES
Three-Part Breathing

Three-part breathing ensures complete utilization of lung capacity and is extremely useful in managing chronic stress.

Lie on your back with your knees raised, so that the soles of your feet are flat on the floor.

Rest your hands by your sides, and feel yourself settled down into the ground. Alternatively, you could sit on a chair with a backrest, buttocks touching the backrest and back erect.

To begin, exhale fully.

You're going to divide up your inhalation into three parts:

- Belly (abdomen centered on your navel),
- Solar plexus (around your lowest ribs), and
- Chest (middle and upper thorax).

Begin your inhalation by taking 1/3 of your breath deep inside as if it is filling your belly. Feel your abdomen rise as you do. Pause.

Then take 1/3 of your breath into your solar plexus. At this stage you should feel your lower chest expanding. Pause.

Finally, inhale the last 1/3 of your breath right up into your chest. You will get a sensation that the chest is filling up to the top, like filling the petrol tank.

Pause at the top, and then reverse the whole thing. Exhale the air from your upper chest, then your solar plexus, and finally your belly.

When you pause do not forcibly hold your breath. The pause is a comma and not full stop, not even a semicolon. Repeat this for a number of times. For many people, the most difficult part to get is the solar plexus or the lower chest. Try and imagine your ribs expanding out to the sides as you breathe into them. When done correctly the belly rises UP, the ribs move OUT, and the upper chest expands upwards. The breathing apparatus expands in all three dimensions.

Three-part breathing needs a lot of practice to master. You have to be patient and aware of your breathing all the time. This type of breathing should be avoided after a meal or when you are completely exhausted.

EXERCISE AND BREATHING

Exercise puts a lot of demands on the cardio-respiratory system. Though aerobic training is often called cardio workout, we must not forget the role of the respiratory system.

During vigorous exercise, oxygen consumption requirements rise from 300 ml/min at rest to about 3000 ml/min. Carbon dioxide production (requiring exhalation) increases from 240 ml/min to 3000 ml/min. To facilitate this, the depth as well as rate of respiration increases.

Breathing with an open mouth is recommended during strenuous exercise, because it provides less airway resistance than breathing through the nose.

Deeper inhalation provides the oxygen needed by muscles for contraction, the quality of inhalation is important for strength, energy, endurance, and regulation of heart rate and blood pressure.

Complete exhalation is needed to empty the lungs of carbon dioxide and to facilitate deep and powerful inhalations. This is ensured by training the muscles of respiration.

Breathing training can enhance performance more dramatically over the long term. An athlete indulging in endurance events will greatly benefit from well structured breathing exercises. Regular breathing practice can help the sportsperson or athlete maintain optimum stress levels during competition.

BREATHING AS FORM OF MEDITATION

Breathing forms the basic pillar over which many meditation techniques are built. The **Vipassna** form of meditation introduced by Gautam Buddha is a technique where one reaches a transcendental state using breathing as a vehicle.

Sakshi Bhava is the ancient way of witnessing one's own mind and ultimately coming to terms with it. Our mind is prone to do a lot of wandering, making it difficult to track it completely. Tracking one's breathing is easier and it is more rhythmic and steady. Let us try being aware of the air that goes in and comes out of our system. Let us try and be a *sakshi* or a witness to our breathing cycle.

CHAPTER 9 : DEEP BREATHING

How do we do this?

Sit with eyes closed on floor or on a chair.

Feel the cool air touch the nostrils as it passes through the throat and enters the lungs during inhalation.

Feel and appreciate the warm air coming out through the same route as we exhale.

This simple procedure allows us to become more aware of our breathing cycle in its natural form. This also allows us to have some sort of a watch on the mind. We get to witness life passing in and out of us and in doing so become more acutely aware of our senses. The thought processes also get streamlined in this way making it easier for us to slip into the Sakshi Bhava.

This watching of the breathing process is, perhaps, the first step of the famous Vipassana meditation, popularized in modern times by the ex-industrialist Sri S N Goenka who got wonderful benefits from this method.

In yogic practices *pranayama* offers a variety of breathing practices to energize, cleanse, soothe and reach higher levels of awareness.

DEEP BREATHING: A QUICK FIX AGAINST STRESS

While performing a hip operation during my orthopaedic training, I encountered torrential bleeding in the surgical wound. As I tried to find the source, rather unsuccessfully, there was lot of panic and even more bleeding. Ultimately I had to call my tutor Dr Shahrookh Vatchha to bail me out. When Dr Vatchha joined me there was blood spurting all over. He asked me to calm down and even suggested that I start singing. As far as he was concerned, he first took a few deep breaths. He then asked for a fresh surgical mop and applied pressure on the wound. For the next five minutes there was no talk. All I could observe was that Dr Vatchha was breathing deeply and grinning. After what felt like eternity, he removed the mop and there was the bleeding blood vessel waiting to be caught and dealt with. Deep breathing helped us drive away the panic situation and the bleeding could be stopped with proactive surgical steps. From that day onwards I was convinced that a few deep breaths can evaporate stress in most cases in an instant.

"Breathe. Let go. And remind yourself that this very moment is the only one you know you have for sure." Oprah Winfrey

> Deep breathing exercises, while providing the body with rich oxygen and ridding of the toxins, are the simplest form of stress busters. Breath awareness can be a very effective form of meditation by itself.

CHAPTER 10

Progressive Muscle Relaxation

The time to relax is when you don't have time for it — Attributed to both Jim Goodwin and Sydney J. Harris

WHAT IS RELAXATION?
According to the Oxford dictionary, relaxing means getting to a state which is less tense or tight. So relaxation is basically an action that involves letting go or releasing.

Progressive Muscle Relaxation therefore is a process wherein the muscle tension is reduced and mental tension is slowly eased out. A relaxed person is one whose heart beat rate is normal, his breathing is slow and deep, there is very little tension in the muscles and the posture is balanced. A relaxed person has a calm expression on the face and his speech is not marred by agitation.

THE IMPORTANCE OF RELAXATION
Relaxation is one of the fundamentals of happiness.

Bliss cannot be achieved without a harmonious mind-body relationship. Relaxation creates a harmonious mind-body relationship and thus it is a prophylaxis and therapy for stress. It's a very potent antidote to the mental and physical effects of stress.

As we have seen earlier, stress today is surfacing as a leading cause of mental anguish

Spare the Thought and Relax
Baba Calm Dev

in many people, leading to countless health problems. These are termed as psychosomatic illnesses.

It all begins with worry and continued mental chatter, which leads to release of stress hormones. The body, under the influence of these hormones responds adversely. Rapid shallow breathing, palpitation and muscle tenseness are the visible effects. Relaxation aims at slowing the breathing, making it deep and rhythmic. Relaxation helps in slowing the resting of heartbeat. The mind focuses on the present activity, thereby reducing the irrelevant mental chatter. Relaxation eases the muscle tension, giving way to a blissful mind-body equation.

Most relaxation techniques aim towards easing out tension in the body and the mind. During acute stress our mind begins to work haphazardly and becomes incapable of coherent, logical and meaningful thought process that can see us through these stressful times. We constantly worry about the future or brood over the past, essentially the mistakes we have made.

However, with the help of relaxation techniques, we are able to attain a calm state of mind which is signified by clarity of thoughts and actions. It also forces us to live life in the moment, something we become incapable of during stress. Relaxation techniques goad us and make us feel vibrant and strong enough to take coercive action against the stressor. From the standpoint of mental and physical well being, relaxation techniques are very important and justifiably so.

RELAXATION AND PERFORMANCE

Whether it is sport or business, the best results are obtained when one is relaxed. A calm mind can function better under duress since it promotes clarity of thought and action. Any top golfer will tell you that winning a major tournament requires as much stress management as a course management. When you want the ball to fall in the hole, a tensed mind can be your enemy. If your mind is worried about the result, you cannot win. A calm, relaxed mind, focused on the game has more chance of success than a mind that is agitated.

CHAPTER 10 : PROGRESSIVE MUSCLE RELAXATION

In most sports, be it golf, cricket, tennis or billiards, a swing, stroke or cueing action needs to be completed. Anxiety and worry stops the swing before completion. A skulled ball in golf, a dropped catch in cricket, a service fault in tennis and a miscue in billiards can all arise out of mental tension. Relaxation ensures that you remain 'in the moment', till the swing is completed, without worrying about the future, here winning the game.

Likewise, in business people lose their cool very often and with it often the deal. Many poor decisions are made in an agitated state, when one is in a reactive mode. A relaxed mind can help you become more proactive and focused, without letting the situation get the better of you. Relaxation helps you douse the fire of stress whose smoke can often suffocate the mind.

HOW TO RELAX?

A lot of stress is created in an effort to relax, says Baba Calm Dev.

True. The very act of trying to relax can produce maximum stress because the body and the mind have little understanding of what they have to achieve. Till what point do they have to let go to be able to truly relax, this is the question that is uppermost in the mind.

To achieve relaxation is a tough proposition. Whenever I perform arthroscopic surgery of the knee under local anesthesia, I want my patient to be in a stage of mental and muscular relaxation. This facilitates easy administration of the local anesthetic around the knee and smooth surgery thereafter.

Most patients are nervous, often petrified when they enter the operation theatre. They see several masked individuals walking around in silence. The temperatures are freezing and the thought of needles and injections is unnerving.

In this scenario when I tell the patient to relax, I usually get him or her more knotted up. I coax some more...

"Please relax... Just try and relax".

"Doctor, I am trying my best" says the patient and would hold his limbs more rigidly.

"No, no keep the leg as loose as possible".

"Is this OK?"

"No, no less tight"...

This would be the flow of conservation for the next few minutes leading to loss of time and an increase in stress within the patient. At this juncture it would be pertinent to relate a story from Baba Calm Dev's repertoire of stories.

A man rings up his neighbour's wife: "Will you come out with me alone tonight?"

"Are you crazy? What do you think I am? If I tell my husband he will kill you." She shouts.

"Don't worry. I am just trying to obey your dear husband."

"What do you mean?"

"Yesterday he threatened to shoot me if I did not stop flirting with you. How can I stop flirting without starting? So will you come out?"

Baba Calm Dev's story comes handy in understanding the Art of Relaxation. Something that needs to stop, first needs to get started. Similarly a body that must relax must first be in a state of tension. This is the most cardinal of all rules.

To create instant relaxation The Stop-Tense formula has been found to really work. I ask the patient to first tense his thigh muscle and hold it really tight. The patient easily responds to the command to tense or contract the muscle. Then I tell him to un-tense, let go... This makes him relax. 'Un-Tense' is a command that is easier than a command to 'Relax'.

PROGRESSIVE MUSCLE RELAXATION

Progressive Muscle Relaxation or PMR is a technique of stress management developed by American physician Edmund Jacobson in the early 1920s. Jacobson argued that since muscular tightness accompanies stress, one can reduce anxiety by learning how to relax the muscles.

Muscle tension produced by mental stress is a psycho-somatic phenomenon. Reduction of mental stress by relaxing the body is

CHAPTER 10 : PROGRESSIVE MUSCLE RELAXATION

somato-psychic in nature and promotes all round relaxation.

Jacobson trained his patients to voluntarily relax certain muscles in their body in order to reduce anxiety symptoms. He also found that relaxation procedures are effective in treating people with peptic ulcers, insomnia, and hypertension. The term 'progressive' denotes the systematic order in which the muscles are tensed and relaxed.

Jacobson's Progressive Relaxation is still popular with modern physical therapists and is used in providing relaxation for professional sportspersons.

BASIC STEPS FOR RELAXATION

Position yourself in a comfortable position. Sit in a comfortable reclining arm chair or lie down on a bed or on a mat on the floor. Your entire body, including your head, should be supported. Lying down on a sofa or bed or sitting in a reclining chair are two ways of supporting your body most completely. When lying down, you may want to place a pillow beneath your knees for further support, as this helps you rest your lumbar spine against the floor. Sitting up is preferable to lying down if you are feeling tired and sleepy. It's advantageous to experience the full depth of the relaxation response consciously without going to sleep.

Wear loose clothes; remove your shoes and get as comfortable as possible. Take off your shoes, watch, glasses, contact lenses, jewellery, and so on.

Select a place where you are least likely to be disturbed. Switch off your cell phone and switch on the air conditioner, if you have one, to block external sounds. Alternatively, you could put on some soft music. Avoid any music with too much of rhythm or else you might get in the 'groove' and jerk while contracting and relaxing.

If you are seated see that your back is well supported. If you are lying down, lie on your back with arms by your side. Do not cross your legs.

The session starts with deep breathing. Take a long deep breath and feel your abdomen rising with inhalation of air. Take a few deep breaths slowly and establish a good breathing rhythm.

Alternately contract and un-tense specific groups of muscles. After the contraction, a muscle will be more relaxed or flaccid than prior to the tensing. Focus your awareness on the muscles, specifically the contrast between tension and relaxation. Be aware of the tension and the relaxation which follows in your muscles. In time, you will recognize tension in any specific muscle and be able to reduce that tension.

Inhale during the contraction and exhale during the relaxation phase. Count up to ten as you inhale. And when you exhale, give the command "let go..." to the muscles.

Note that each step is really two steps, one cycle of tension-relaxation for each set of opposing muscles.

Practise at least 20 minutes per day. You could do two sessions initially, when you are getting the hang of it. Once a day is mandatory for obtaining optimum effect.

As you become an expert in relaxation technique, you will find that the amount of time you need to experience the relaxation response will decrease.

SOME DON'TS THAT ARE TO BE FOLLOWED

Don't tense muscles other than the specific group at each step.

Don't hold your breath, grit your teeth, or squint. Breathe slowly and evenly and think only about the tension-relaxation contrast.

PMR should not be performed on a full stomach. Food digestion after meals will tend to disrupt deep relaxation.

Each tensing is for 10 seconds; each relaxing is for 10 or 15 seconds. Do not take on more than this.

Do the entire sequence once a day until you feel you are able to control your muscle tensions. If you have any health problems, consult your doctor first.

PMR starts from your fingers and ends with your toes. From the fingers and hands you go progressively upwards to your forearms, arms, shoulders, neck and face. You then go lower from the chest,

CHAPTER 10 : PROGRESSIVE MUSCLE RELAXATION

back, hips, thighs, knees, calves, feet and finally the toes. Keeping a fixed progress of regions ensures that you do not miss any part.

THE 16-STEP PMR
1. Hands
Clench your fists on inhalation. On exhalation extend or straighten the fingers and let go.

2. Wrists
Flex your wrist and feel tension in the front of the forearm, then let go. Extend the wrist to feel contraction on the back of the forearm, then relax.

3. Arms
Tense the biceps; let go, and drop your arm by your side. The triceps are tensed by trying to hyper-extend the elbow and relax.

4. Shoulders
Raise your arms high up trying to reach the ceiling and then flop them down. If you are seated, rotate your shoulders as if you are scratching your back and then let go.

5. Neck (side turn)
With the shoulders straight and relaxed, turn the head slowly to the right, as far as you can; relax. Turn to the left; relax.

6. Neck (forward bend)
Dig your chin into your chest; relax. Gently extend your neck by looking upward and then relax.

7. Mouth
Open your mouth as far as possible; then relax. Bring your lips together till they are pursed as tightly as possible; then relax.

8. Tongue
Dig your tongue into the roof of your mouth; relax. Dig it into the bottom of your mouth; relax.

9. Eyes
Open them as wide as possible (furrow your brow); relax. Close your eyes tightly and then relax. Make sure you completely relax the eyes, forehead, and nose after each of the contractions.

10. Upper back
Pull your shoulders back or retract them to feel the tension in the upper back and then relax. Push the shoulders forward or protract them to hunch then let go.

11. Abdomen
Pull in the stomach as far as possible; relax completely. Push out the stomach or tense it as if you were preparing for a punch in the gut; relax.

12. Back
With shoulders resting on the back of the chair, push your body forward so that your back is arched; relax. Be very careful with this one, or don't do it at all.

13. Butt
Tense the butt tightly and raise pelvis slightly off chair; relax. Dig buttocks into chair; relax.

14. Thighs
Raise your legs about 6 inches off the floor or the foot rest; relax. Dig your heels into the floor or foot rest; relax.

15. Calves and feet
Point the toes downwards without raising the legs; relax. Point the feet up as far as possible; relax.

CHAPTER 10 : PROGRESSIVE MUSCLE RELAXATION

16. Toes
With legs relaxed, dig your toes into the floor; relax. Bend the toes up as far as possible; relax.

Now just relax for a while. Continue to breathe deep and enjoy the relaxed sensation.

With more practice, you may wish to skip the steps that do not appear to be a problem for you. In a few weeks after you've understood which areas need more work, you will be able to make more progress. You can now move to a shortened procedure where your entire body will be relaxed.

As you reduce the tension you carry in your body, your whole being will feel less stressed out and you will enjoy increased physical and emotional health. These exercises will not eliminate stress, but when it arises, you will know it immediately, and you will be able to cope with it in a better way than most others.

However, there are certain things to keep in mind to ensure that you benefit the most from your relaxation techniques. First, make a decision not to worry about anything. Give yourself permission to put aside the concerns of the day. Allow taking care of yourself and having peace of mind to take precedence over any of your worries. Success with relaxation depends on giving high priority to your peace of mind in your overall scheme of things.

Secondly, assume a passive, detached attitude. This is probably the most important element. Do not try too hard to relax. Do not try to control your body. Do not judge your performance. The moot point here is to let go.

IMPROVE YOUR AXE FACTOR
You may have heard about the two woodcutters who were working relentlessly to chop down timber. One of them was so committed that he hardly took a break. The other took frequent breaks and yet chopped more wood than his friend.

What was he doing in these breaks?

He was sharpening his axe.

CALM SUTRA : THE ART OF RELAXATION

Moral of the story: Take a break. Relax. Sharpen your senses.

"Relaxation improves your AXE factor", says Baba Calm Dev.

> The mind and body can be relaxed by releasing tension from the muscles. This is easily done by following the "Stop-Tense" formula. In this method, after tensing the muscle, a simple command of "Let-go" achieves relaxation.

The Postures of Calm Sutra

CHAPTER 11

Bad posture can cause stress, just as stress can cause bad posture. The Calm Sutra recommends good posture as a prime way to get a hold on your stress with great health benefits.

Posture, also known as physical alignment or form, denotes the position and alignment of the body during various activities like sleeping, sitting, standing, walking, lifting, playing and exercising. Posture is the way a person chooses to keep his limbs, head and torso together so as to keep the body balanced and steady.

Basically posture refers to the positioning of various body parts with respect to the ever-present force of gravity. Whether we are standing, sitting or lying down; gravity exerts a force on our joints, ligaments and muscles. Good posture entails distributing the force of gravity through our body so that no one structure is overstressed.

Very often attitude of mind and posture of body are closely related. A stressed mind could cause a faulty posture of the body and vice-versa.

Having a good posture is very important because it allows you to breathe properly. With hunched shoulders, the volume of your chest cavity is reduced and limits your ability to take deep breaths. Even a small slouch can

> Postures are vital in Calm Sutra. Your pose can expose you
> *Baba Calm Dev*

cause you to have shallow breathing which is not required when in crisis.

It is possible to guess a person's mental make-up and attitude by looking at the posture of his body. This has been termed as body language and used to read people during important social interactions like job interviews. A good posture can make you feel healthy and happy and eradicate much of the medical and orthopaedic problems.

DEVELOPMENT OF POSTURE

Postures probably have their genesis in very early childhood, in the infant stage to be precise. The child at this stage starts imitating a parent or a role model and develops a certain style of standing or walking which is akin to that of his parents. This grows into a habit.

During the adolescent years, postures, gait, style are often aped from popular idols. The adolescent may slouch just to look cool and hip. A teenage girl conscious of her growing breasts, slouches her shoulders to conceal or underplay her maturity. Some boys develop a swagger and others may stick out their chest. Slowly, what started out as fun gets incorporated into one's personality and in this way, faulty postures do stick on. Faulty postures create tensions in certain groups of muscles, which could result in permanent imbalance in muscles. Hence it is imperative to get children to have a good body posture right from the start. For this parents need to improve their postures too if they have to be good role models for their children.

CAN FAULTY POSTURE CAUSE HARM?

Many orthopaedic disorders are associated with poor posture. Back and neck problems head the list. Knee pains, muscle soreness, fatigue and even headaches are commonly seen. Faulty posture results in alteration of biomechanics in the various joints in the body. Faulty posture causes muscle imbalance and abnormal transfer of body weight, which can have disastrous consequences. A slouch can cause contraction of the flexor muscles and stretching of the extensor muscles of the back. Over the years this can develop into a permanent bony deformity and cause chronic backache. Persons using a faulty

CHAPTER 11 : THE POSTURES OF CALM SUTRA

pillow while sleeping can invite problems of the cervical spine with spasms and stiffness of various muscles of the neck.

Persons engaged in sitting for prolonged periods on chairs, which are too low for them, cause excessive flexion of the knee joint and subsequent knee pains. Orthopaedic conditions like spondylosis and knee osteoarthritis can be traced back to poor attitudes of the body.

Contorted facial expressions like continuous frowning can cause excruciating headaches due to continuous muscle tightness.

CORRECT POSTURE: AN IN-DEPTH DISCOURSE

A person has correct posture if he stands, sits, and sleeps, in a relaxed position while keeping his muscles relaxed and joints at optimum position. The body should be aligned properly and the spine should not deviate abnormally. The alignment of the body should be as linear as possible without deviations. There should be no crouches or slouches.

In a Nutshell, a Good Posture Ought to Include:

- A straight line from your ears, shoulders, hips, knees and ankles
- Centered head
- Shoulders, hips and knees at equal height
- No leaning forward of the head
- Squared and not rounded shoulders
- The back should not be arched
- Avoid an excessive posterior pelvic tilt (protruding backside)
- Avoid an excessive anterior pelvic tilt (protruding abdomen/pelvis).

A GOOD STANDING POSTURE

For a correct and comfortable standing posture, the width of your stance should be as much as the breadth of your shoulders. This distributes your body weight evenly and gives you better balance.

The position of your lower back is very important, while standing. Very often, one tends to create an excessive extension of the lower spine. This posture makes the tummy jut out more and puts excessive stress on the back. Prolonged standing with the spine extended can reduce the efficiency of the abdominal muscles and weaken them. A good idea is to slightly tuck in the tummy, without much tension, and the spine will straighten out.

The chest should be in the same line as the pelvis when viewed from the side. This reduces the chances of slouching. The shoulders should not droop but should be as square as possible. Head is to be held high without any deviations in the neck. The ideal standing posture creates maximum distance between the head and the toes and avoids any lateral deviations.

The body should be as relaxed as possible. To practiSe correct standing, stand with your back touching the wall *(refer to the wall test described later in this chapter)*.

When standing, proper posture involves aligning the body correctly, so that the pull of gravity is evenly distributed.

A GOOD SITTING POSTURE

One ought to choose his chair correctly. This involves a special knowledge of the science of ergonomics. Height and occupation are two important factors to be considered while choosing a chair. A good chair for a six-footer may not suit a person who is 5 feet 5 inches. A person who is on a computer needs a chair different from the one who is a telephone operator. Today job-specific chairs are available. While choosing a chair, see that the height of the chair seat, reaches just below your knees. When you sit with your shoulders relaxed, your elbows should rest comfortably on the arm rests. See that your lower back is well supported and most of your thighs are supported by the seat. You should not be flexing your knees too much or struggling to reach the ground. The lower back should not slide away from the backrest and your shoulders should not droop to reach the armrests. Remember that many of us spend more than eight hours on a chair and it is worthwhile to spend some time on selecting the right chair.

There are a lot of people who use the computer these days for

CHAPTER 11 : THE POSTURES OF CALM SUTRA

long stretches of time. Often it leads to a host of pains and stress areas because people do not follow proper postural guidelines.

I have compiled some guidelines to be kept in mind **for those who work for long in front of the computer**.

- Make sure your chair is comfortable and adjusted to your height and limb length.
- Sit in a position so that your pelvis is upright and try and ensure your thighs are at a 110 degree angle to your trunk.
- Ensure the lumbar support of your chair fits the small of your back so that it maintains the natural 'S' shape of your spine. Buttocks should touch the backrest.
- The armrests of the chair should touch your forearms, when your shoulders and elbows are relaxed at your side. This helps to avoid strain in your neck and upper limbs.
- Also, make sure there is adequate thigh support whilst allowing movement without obstruction.
- Make full use of the chair movement especially when reaching for items such as the phone.
- Avoid slouching and alter your position frequently when using a keyboard.
- Change your posture frequently to give your muscles a break, and remember to take frequent breaks from your desk.
- Keep your mouse and telephone as close as possible allowing you to remain relaxed and in a natural position at your desk.
- Ensure your monitor is square on so you don't have to turn your head to look at it.
- Adjust your screen so that it is at arm's length away from your face and the top of the screen is horizontal to your eye line.

GOOD SLEEPING POSTURE

For a good sleeping posture, the pillow and the mattress should be firm, giving your body good and adequate support without allowing your body to sink in them. The pillow should ideally extend from the shoulder blades to the top of the head. This ensures that the neck is neither flexed nor extended excessively. The pillow should be thick enough to provide the natural curve of the cervical spine comfortable support. If you habitually sleep on your side then the pillows should be as thick as the distance between your ear and the tip of your shoulder to ensure that your cervical spine is not bent sideways.

Generally speaking, a supine posture (on the back) is considered an ideal sleeping posture. To relax your lower back you could place a small pillow under your calves. When the knees are flexed, the lumbar spine is rested. Unfortunately, the sleeping posture is not within our control once sleep sets in, but let there be a good beginning at least.

WALKING RIGHT

The key word to correct walking is to walk straight and walk tall. There are two aspects of correct walking. One aspect is related to the body posture and the second aspect relates to the foot mechanics that come into play while walking.

The body posture should be as erect as possible while walking. As with standing, the walk should also avoid any deviations of the torso. Get the feeling of elongating the body while walking. Hold your head high, keep shoulders wide, tuck your tummy in, and swing your arms naturally without any tension. When you stride you should get the feeling that your feet are elongating your entire lower extremity and making your stride optimally long.

The foot mechanics are very important while walking. The heel should strike the ground first, then the rest of the foot bears the weight of the body and finally the front of the foot propels you forwards. If these little things are kept in mind, one can develop a healthy walk that is high on grace too.

LIFTING THINGS CORRECTLY

Dynamic posture or form deals with performing actions correctly with minimal risks to your musculo-skeletal system. One of the frequent activities, which could cause damage to your back, is lifting things up from ground level. Whether you are lifting a one-year-old child or a suitcase, you have to be careful while executing

CHAPTER 11 : THE POSTURES OF CALM SUTRA

the action else you might end up with a sore back, a crick in the neck or worse, with a slipped disc that can be very painful and keep you out of action for a long time.

There are two points that one must keep in mind while lifting things from the ground level. Bend at your knees, rather than bending from your back to pick up things. The quadriceps muscles, which help you lift weights while straightening out your knees, are stronger than your back muscles. The knees are more adept at lifting weights than your delicate spinal joints. This makes squatting while lifting far safer and more effective than bending your back.

Hold the object close to your body. Unless you are lifting something very hot it is better to lift objects close to your body. This reduces the load moment on your spinal joints. It is easier to lift a child close to you rather than with your arms extended. Remember to bend your elbows while lifting objects. This will automatically ensure that the load is close to the axis of your body.

AWARENESS AND ACTION FOR GOOD POSTURE
How does one know if one's posture is right or not.

Awareness: (Test Your Posture)
To figure out if you have good posture, take the following posture tests.

The Wall Test - Stand with the back of your head touching the wall and your heels six inches from the baseboard. With your buttocks touching the wall, stick your hand between your lower back and the wall, and then between your neck and the wall. If you can get within an inch or two at the low back and two inches at the neck, you are close to having excellent posture.

The Mirror Test - Stand facing a full length mirror and check to see if:
- Your head is straight
- Your shoulders are level
- Your hips are level
- Your kneecaps face the front

- Your ankles are straight

Have someone else check you out for the following:
- Your head is held straight and not slumped
- Chin is parallel to the floor
- Shoulders are in line with ears
- Knees are straight
- Slight forward curve to your lower back

Action:
Once we are aware of the faults in our posture, we can take remedial action. The self-replicating vicious cycle of stress-posture-stress is reversible through relaxation. A deep breath and corrective action is all that is required. When you are in front of the computer, take periodical rests and widen your arms and swing it around a bit. Remember the classic pose in the movie *Titanic*? Do something like that and you are bound to feel rejuvenated.

After a week or two of awareness and proper action, you will begin to discover that your back and shoulders are not as tense as they used to be. As you continue to practice, you will realize that even under stress your body remains relaxed. You may then notice others respond to your relaxed body differently since by then your entire body language would have changed for the better.

> Good posture is essential for good health. Sitting, standing, sleeping, walking and lifting correctly can help us avoid a host of orthopaedic problems, as well as beat stress. Good posture also improves the "outer you" adding grace to your body language.

Meditation

CHAPTER 12

A conversation with Baba Calm Dev

Baba: "Who are You?"

Me: "I am Dilip Nadkarni."

B: "Oh, that's the name given to you by your parents. Who are you?"

M: "I am a man, 179 cm, 82 kg... "

B: "That's your sex, height and weight. That's not you."

M: "I am an orthopaedic surgeon, son of Geeta and Vasant Nadkarni, husband of Rashmi, father of Nishad and Rishab, staying at..."

B: "That's your profession, your relationship with people and your address, but not you."

M: "I am my mind, my thoughts..."

B: "You are close, but that's still not you..."

You are not your body, you are not your mind, and you are not even your thoughts.

You are just consciousness. You are pure awareness.

You are not your mind because you can be aware of the mind.

You are not your thought because you can be aware of your thought.

You are thus distinct from your body, your mind and your thought.

You are the consciousness, which feels and witnesses everything as life progresses.

This pure awareness or consciousness is the real 'You' - peaceful and calm and meditation is the process to know this consciousness within you.

> Meditation purifies your Atmasphere.
> *Baba Calm Dev*

Baba then asked me to sit quietly and observe my breath.

I sat quietly observing my breathing. I could feel the breath enter my body, as I inhaled. I could feel the air leave my body as I exhaled. I consciously took long, deep breaths. I was already feeling good. However my mind still had a lot of thoughts. Had the operated patient been shifted to the room? This was my first thought. I brushed it aside and resumed my attention to the breathing.

Again I was disturbed by another thought. Had the cheque been realized? I fought to regain my concentration. Breathe, I told myself. I returned to the present and continued my breathing. I continued sitting and breathing. A golf game outcome crossed my mind, but I persisted. I opened my eyes after what seemed to be 10 minutes. Baba had gone, but I had met the owner of my mind. I was aware of the consciousness, which was distinct from my thoughts. Was this meditation?

WHAT IS MEDITATION?

The word meditation is derived from two Latin words: *Meditari* which means to think, dwell upon and exercise the mind and *Mederi* which means to heal. Its Sanskrit derivation *medha* means wisdom.

There are many definitions and descriptions of meditation. However the more practical definition in the modern scenario would be:

Meditation is a practice of conscious or mindful focus upon a sound, an object, the breath, body movement or thought, in order to increase awareness of the present moment, reduce stress, promote relaxation, and enhance personal and spiritual growth.

Meditation has been mystified by Godmen. It has been made to sound almost unattainable to mere mortals. Classic scriptures have stated that to attain true states of meditation one must go through several stages of spiritual evolution. Meditation has been associated with penance, austerity, physical hardship and concentrated contemplation to attain a union with divinity. The process has been described to be hard and one has to leave worldly passions and

CHAPTER 12 : MEDITATION

desires if one wants to get enlightenment through meditation. Union with the eternal truth, Moksha and Nirvana have been offered as the proclaimed end points of successful meditation.

To me meditation means awareness. Whatever you do with awareness is meditation. Watching your breath mindfully is meditation. Listening to the birds is meditation. Swimming, walking or playing golf with awareness is meditation. The criterion is that these activities should be free from any other distraction to the mind. One need not sit in an exaggerated lotus posture, which in all probability could damage your knees, to meditate. The Himalayas are not the only place where meditation happens. It can be done in the comforts of one's room. Music and dance are also considered forms of meditation since these activities go on to relax your mind and improve your health. They help you connect with the Supreme Power and attain joy and fulfillment.

ACCIDENTAL MEDITATION

Many times by accident we achieve an almost thought-free mind. Like when we sing a melody and our voice pitches in with the musical instrument, the words in sync with the beat. The entire experience, that is so exhilarating, can be described as a meditative state.

Again during a game of table tennis there are occasions where there are no thoughts, a somewhat 'no mind zone'. During rallies, there are no thoughts that flit across. Only actions. When the rally is over, you notice that you were completely immersed in the task, totally thought free and ecstatic... A trance like meditative state.

MY EXPOSURE TO MEDITATION

Born into a Chitrapur Saraswat Brahmin family, I was exposed to meditation early in life. A thread ceremony was performed where my father whispered the *Gayatri Mantra* in my ear. The *Gayatri Mantra* is a set of words in Sanskrit to be chanted in the mind. After the thread ceremony I memorized the mantra and religiously did the *sandhi* or *sandhya vandan*, the ritual of chanting the mantra. At the age of ten, I did not relish the meditative aspect of the mantra, but did it as a matter of routine. One of my favourite uncles, Savanal Ganeshmam would aid me in my routine. He would state, "No *sandhi*, no chocolate" and ensure that I performed the *sandhya vandan*. The ritual of mantra chanting continued for a month and thereafter the frequency dropped. The mantra was mainly chanted by me, before going for an exam or before a table-tennis match. It really helped me during testing times. That was my initiation into meditation.

My second exposure to meditation came during my visit to the Rajneesh ashram. All my concepts of meditation were restructured by the Maestro. My idea of meditation was sitting cross-legged at the altar and chanting the *Gayatri Mantra* under my breath. At the Ashram, meditation was anything but that. I was exposed to a new form of meditation which required us to utter gibberish, twirl around like possessed dervishes. The ashram techniques included laughing, crying, dancing, screaming and celebrating; all this interspersed with complete silence. The experience was a complete catharsis for the emotional garbage that I had been carrying all this while.

In recent times I have found a variety of activities, which transport me into the path of meditation. I get great gratification with the combination of deep breathing and music or the *swar* meditation.

My brushes with meditation continued with my Guruji Shrimat Sadyojat Shankarashrama who bestowed on me a mantra and set me on journey to find my inward self.

I took to a gamut of physical activities like table tennis, athletics, weight lifting, walking, jogging and golf. The later opened up a new vista for me as it is a near ideal form of meditation for me. Deep breathing, focused awareness of the green surroundings, the strategies...all help to make golf one of the most relaxing and meditative forms of experience.

TYPES OF MEDITATION:
There are many types of meditation one can choose from.

CHAPTER 12 : MEDITATION

Meditation ranges from quiet introspection to loud chanting of mantras. From deep breathing to dancing like a possessed; from Vipassana to Dynamic Dancing; from Yoganidra to putting on the golf course...you can choose one or go in for a combination of meditative forms. The best way to choose your style is by trying out what works for you. Meditation is a hands-on phenomenon where no one can help out. It is you and you alone who can decide what suits you the most and proceed accordingly. Like you have to jump into the water in order to learn how to swim, so also you have to experience meditation yourself.

Transcendental Meditation (TM)

Maharishi Mahesh Yogi introduced **Transcendental Meditation** to the Western world. TM is by far the most thoroughly researched meditation technique in terms of its benefits for mental, physical, and social health. Since 1958, 4 million people have learned TM, including celebrities like the Beatles, Arnold Schwarzenegger, Sylvester Stallone and several international sportsmen and industry leaders. Over five hundred scientific studies have been conducted on TM at more than two hundred universities worldwide and established it as a holistic form of healthcare. This practical, proven meditation procedure requires no special skills or a drastic change of lifestyle. TM is voted by many as the most effective stress buster available to gain deep relaxation, promote good health, increase creativity and attain inner happiness and fulfillment.

Transcendental Meditation is an easy to learn, enjoyable practice that enriches all areas of life.

The Meditation technique is a form of meditation, practiced 20 minutes twice a day, sitting comfortably with the eyes closed. It is essential that you learn TM from a certified trainer. The instructor gives you a special phrase or mantra. This mantra is to be kept as a secret and never to be divulged. You are told to repeat the mantra over and over again silently.

While meditating if distracting thoughts pop up, you're instructed to simply observe them. Do not follow them or try to force them out.

Having observed the thought, gently return your mental focus to your personal mantra.

Many scientific studies have established that the mind assumes deep relaxation with TM. There is Electro-encephalogram (EEG) evidence to support this claim. TM has also documented increased intelligence, more creativity and contentment in life. Russian researchers have shown that TM can induce unique activity patterns in the brain creating a state of "restful alertness". Alcoholism and drug addiction have been shown to reverse with TM. Objective decrease of blood pressure and other stress related illnesses makes TM an authentic technique to reduce psycho-somatic problems.

Vipassana

Vipassana is an ancient Buddhist technique of meditation, which means to see things as they really are. Vipassana is sometimes called mindfulness or insight meditation. It is the art of becoming deeply aware of the present moment. Mindfulness is the practice of being aware of what is happening here and now. I have been fortunate to have attended a short workshop on Vipassana by its current teacher Mr. Satya Narayan Goenka.

Mr. Goenka was born and raised in Myanmar, where he learnt Vipassana from his teacher, Sayagyi U Ba Khin. Mr. Goenka received training in the meditation technique from his teacher for fourteen years, before settling down in India in 1969. His headquarters in India are at Igatpuri, where 10 day residential courses are conducted free of cost. Mr. Goenka, over the years has imparted the technique to thousands of people, belonging to different races and religion in both the East and the West.

In 1982 he began to appoint assistant teachers to help him meet the growing demand for Vipassana courses. Children and teenagers can be initiated into Vipassana through shorter courses. Vipassana Courses are even being conducted in prisons, which have changed the behavioural pattern of the inmates and jailers alike. It was actually found that inmates who completed the 10-day course were less violent than other inmates

CHAPTER 12 : MEDITATION

The programme is rigourous and requires hard, serious work. No participant is allowed to leave midway and has to complete the course. Activities like reading, writing and talking are forbidden. Men and women are segregated throughout the course. The food consists of a delicious vegetarian lunch at 11.30 am after which, there is nothing but tea and fruits at 5 pm. Meditation continues virtually nonstop through the day, save for a few breaks for food and calls of nature, demanding very high levels of self-control and concentration.

There are three steps to the training.
- The first step is to establish a code of moral conduct, where one abstains from thoughts of killing, stealing, sex and falsehood. This calms the mind and prepares it to perform the task of self-observation.
- The next step is to develop some control over the mind by learning to focus one's attention on the flow of breath as it enters and leaves the nostrils. By the fourth day the mind is more calm and in a position to observe sensations throughout the body. The mind is now harnessed to the task of studying the subtle sensations within the body like heat, cold, pain, itching and throbbing.
- In the final stage the students learn to impart kindness and share goodwill towards all beings. On the tenth day, the silence ends and the participants are finally allowed to talk.

A few of my friends who have completed the course have experienced a visible change in their outlook towards life. We too have found them to be much more easygoing and compassionate after the 10-day Vipassana course. Many of them have revisited Igatpuri to gain more proficiency in the art of Vipassana.

Dynamic Meditation
Though active meditation or dynamic meditation has been largely popularized by Rajneesh and the Osho communion, it has existed over centuries and pointers towards its existence come from books and historical documents. The practice of whirling or spinning while

in a meditative trance originated among the Turkish Sufis. It is still practised by Sufis the world over and dervishes aim to reach *kemal* or the perfect through this dance form that is a highest form of meditation.

Another form of divine dynamic meditation, which is seen in India, is followed by the members of the Varkari group. The energetic dance of the Varkari pilgrims has been in existence for a long time. The Varkari pilgrims of Maharashtra in India, dance their way to the Vithoba temple in Pandharpur. For the Varkari, the dance is out of religious ecstasy and fervour in the anticipation of getting a *darshan* of their deity. The Varkari is instructed to sing and dance with gay abandon on his way to bliss. No Varkari ever returns home without shedding his or her anxieties and stress.

Dynamic Meditation and My Personal Experience

The fascinating Dynamic Meditation, which I attended, was at the Rajneesh Ashram in Pune. It was a divine experience and on a beautiful chilly December morning, we plunged into Dynamic Meditation. The meditation was performed in five stages.

The first stage consisted of breathing rapidly in and out through the nose, concentrating on the exhalation. The breathing had to be deep and chaotic. The second stage consisted of exploding. Getting completely out of control. Going totally mad... Singing, screaming, laughing, shouting, crying, jumping, shaking, dancing and throwing yourself around was allowed. It required holding nothing back, keeping your whole body moving. In the third stage we raised our arms and shouted the mantra Hoo... Hoo...Hoo... from the bottom of our belly. We jumped up and down as we shouted till near exhaustion. In the fourth stage we just froze, assuming any position we desired. At this stage we relaxed completely, being a passive witness to what was happening within. The fifth and the last stage was given to celebration and in tune with music, we danced and celebrated our new found joy and ecstasy.

Dynamic Meditation, though exciting and fascinating, may need some precautions to be safe and effective. As there may be falling

CHAPTER 12 : MEDITATION

or rolling on the ground involved in the meditation, a large room or hall with thick carpeting is needed. Indulging in meditation outdoors, in the early morning, on a soft, well tended lawn would be ideal because the last thing one would want is to be injured while in the throes of such a state.

There are many more varieties of meditation, such the Gazing Meditation, Kundalini Meditation, Tantric Meditation, Zen Meditation and several others. Each has its own set of rules and ways of getting to a state when a person is immersed in his being and experiences a communion with the Supreme Power. These specialized forms of meditation, however, need proper training and mindset for best results.

BENEFITS OF MEDITATION
Meditation Alters the Stress Response
Researchers say that meditation works at least in part by lowering your body's responsiveness to the stress hormone, nor-epinephrine. Normally, stress triggers the release of these hormones, which in turn causes your heart rate, blood pressure and other such vital signs to rise and fluctuate. Meditation interrupts that flow of stress chemicals, and you don't feel knotted or cramped up. In short, when you meditate regularly, you're able to control your body's reaction to stress instead of it controlling you. In a sense it is like a biofeedback technique which allows an individual to monitor and take charge of his own physical reactions to stress.

As we have seen, the list of illnesses exacerbated or aggravated by stress is huge. Meditation has shown to reduce hypertension, heart disease, headaches, anxiety, PMS, sleep disorders and even chronic conditions like rheumatoid arthritis and ankylosing spondylitis. It is also known to help in battling out cancer and other infectious diseases.

Meditation Boosts the Immune System
Research has found that meditation has a favourable action on our immune system. The efficiency of our immune system is essential

if we have to fight a disease. Volunteers who meditated for eight weeks showed a higher level of antibodies in their blood stream than the control group, consisting of those who did not meditate. The state of relaxed awareness brought about by meditation and the boost it gives to the physical system as a whole helps our body and mind repair itself rather fast.

Meditation Increases Creativity and Performance

Meditation improves the performance levels of an individual since it improves concentration, makes the individual open his senses to other aspects of the problem at hand, shortens the reaction time and in general improves the ability to tackle the problem at hand. The right side of our brain are attuned to deal with creative processes and meditation improves this ability in the brain. Creativity, in all art forms such as poetry, music, dance, painting and the likes is shown to improve remarkably with meditation.

Meditation is also known to have assisted sportspersons and helped them in giving in their best. This is because meditation improves physical levels of fitness, boosts immunity, reduces anxiety and makes the person more strong, physically and mentally, to take on his adversaries.

Improves Self-esteem

Increased self awareness, which is one of the features of meditation, improves self esteem. The false ego is discarded to make place for a true sense of self worth.

De-addiction with Meditation

Smoking, alcoholism and even drug addiction have often been eradicated with the help of meditation. Research has shown that people have successfully given up chemical dependence with the help of meditation. There have been fewer cases of relapse in people who have continued the practice of meditation.

CHAPTER 12 : MEDITATION

Meditation is an Antidote for Boredom

The person who meditates has no time for boredom or loneliness and is content with his own company. He does not fear being 'alone' and in fact is able to enjoy his time with himself. He develops a more positive frame of mind and derives enjoyment from his activities and his experiences.

Slows down Aging

Meditation can relieve stress and thereby slow down the degenerative process of the body. Hence ageing process is kept at bay. The factors of aging like blood pressure, eyesight, joint function, hearing etc are better preserved by meditation. Research conducted by University of Pennsylvania has shown promising result of the effect of meditation on Alzheimer's disease, the most obvious malady of premature aging.

THE CALM SUTRA SWAR MEDITATION

I would like to share with you my favourite method of meditation. *Swar* means a musical note. Exhalation of air through our voice box can produce a sound which can be used to soothe. The sound can be used as a focal point of awareness. When this sound reverberates in our body we can reach transcendental heights.

The meditation begins with good posture. If you are fit, healthy and a follower of yoga, sit cross-legged on a mat. Else, if you prefer to sit on a chair, see that your back is well supported. Sit as erect as possible without slouching.

The first step towards this process is to establish an easy relaxed breathing rhythm. Breathe through your nose and exhale through your mouth. After 5 easy breaths, start inhaling more deeply, feeling your belly expanding with each inhalation. At this stage all your attention should be on your breath. Enjoy feeling the air enter deep into your body and feel it slowly go out.

The next step is to create the sound 'Calm' as you are exhaling your breath. There are three distinct syllables to the word calm.

1) Ca (Ka) 2) Aa (aaaa) and 3) Mm (mmmm)

Ca (ka) is generated as you open your mouth. You should feel that the sound is emanated from the belly region. The Ca gives way to Aa (aaaa). The mouth opens more as you say aaaa. Feel the sound rising up the thorax right up to the neck. The last part of Calm ends in Mm (mmmm) and this is said with the mouth closed. The mmmm reverberates in the head area.

Calm, the word if uttered in one flow emanates a sound that arises in the abdomen, reaches the chest and finally culminates as a hum in the head.

If you are musically inclined you could add in a musical note from a keyboard to this mantra of saying CALM. If you listen carefully you can hook on the hum of the air-conditioner or the strains of the *tanpura*. You could buy a CD of a *tanpura* created strain/drone or download the same from our web site www.calmsutra.org.

> Meditation is a practice of conscious or mindful focus upon a sound, an object, the breath, body movement or thought, in order to increase awareness of the present moment, reduce stress, promote relaxation, and enhance personal and spiritual growth. Meditation includes a wide range of activities like deep breathing, chanting, listening to music, dancing and even golf. Meditation improves health in toto.

CHAPTER 13

Meditative Eating

THE JAPANESE TEA CEREMONY

In 1987, I went to Japan to learn Arthroscopic Surgery of the knee joint from the pioneers in this field. Apart from Arthroscopic Surgery, I learnt many more things from the Japanese, essentially about their life, lifestyles, values and principles they live by. I got to see their commitment to science, sincerity to their work, even when they went unsupervised, and their zest for life and its bounties.

A traditional tea ceremony was held in our honour. For me, it was an experience of a lifetime. I was told that the tea ceremony had roots in the 16th century and was created by a Zen priest named Murata Shuko. The ceremony is called *Cha-no-yu*, literally meaning 'hot water tea' and celebrates even the mundane aspects of everyday life.

The Japanese used to have their tea houses away from the main quarters. However, all that has changed in recent times.

The flooring of the room in which we were to be served was done up in wood and very tastefully decorated with hanging scrolls and floral arrangements. The seating was traditionally Japanese, on the floor at a low table. There was soft percussive music in the background.

We were first served a light sweet snack. Taking cue from Hitomi, our local friend, I bowed lightly when I was presented the snack. The selected snack was to be eaten

> Eat using all your senses, with full awareness and you will soon forget what's eating you.
> *Baba Calm Dev*

CALM SUTRA : THE ART OF RELAXATION

with a wooden pick called a *kuromoji*, after it was placed on the special napkin called a *kaishi*.

Our hostess with deliberate graceful movements cleansed and arranged all the tea utensils like the tea bowl, whisk and tea scoop. She then began making the tea, using precise measurements of powdered green tea and water.

The conversation was minimal so that we could enjoy the sights, smells and sounds of the tearoom and the tea-making process.

As I was the guest of honour, the tea bowl was served to me first, which I accepted bowing to the host. There was bowing all around. Hitomi took her bowl and mimed to me about what was to follow.

Before drinking, I had to rotate the bowl, avoiding drinking from the front of the cup. After taking a couple of sips, taking Hitomi's cue I wiped the rim with my fingers, rotated the bowl back, and passed it on to my neighbour with a bow. I wiped my fingers on the *kaishi*.

Once all the guests had been served, the host ritually cleaned the utensils. I did as I was told and examined and admired the utensils. All the others too admired each utensil with respect and gentle care.

At the end of the ceremony, the host and hostess gathered up the utensils and escorted us to the door to bow farewells. To me this was one of the most wonderful experiences of my life and it will always be vivid in my memory for the simplicity with which the Japanese took an ordinary thing like tea making, and turned it into an art form.

EATING WITH AWARENESS: MEDITATIVE EATING

I remember two friends in college with diametrically opposite eating habits. Guru would eat his food at one go. In fact, he would gobble while Suru would savour his food. Guru could finish half a kilo of *bhajiyas*, before you could blink. Hot *bhajiyas*, which could scald normal tongues, had no effect on his. Suru on the other hand would romance his food. He used to take a lot of time eating his lunch. He would sit alone, neatly spread out a newspaper and lay out his *dabba* on it which would contain an assortment of rotis, rice, dal,

CHAPTER 13 : MEDITATIVE EATING

vegetables, a piece of fish and some curd. There was also a small box containing pickle. His lunch was a combination of colours -- yellow dal, green vegetables, brown rotis, white rice... The food would be hot and smell delicious. Suru would sit absorbed in the sights, smells and textures of his food. He would then proceed to eat his food completely immersed in the task. He would chew carefully and enjoy every morsel, without missing out on any of the tastes. He would take his time, drink water intermittently. For Suru lunch was not just a necessary afternoon task to satisfy his hunger. It was an enjoyable event, a form of meditation. From the opening of the *dabba* to polishing off the last spoonful of curds, it was a journey of gastronomic delight.

Suru's partaking of his food and the way the Japanese had their tea had certain remarkable likeness. Both involved all the senses in the appreciation of food, especially the colours, the textures, the tastes, the feelings. Both endeavoured to receiving pleasure from the simple delights of life.

Like my friend Guru, many of us gobble, shovel or chomp on food with our mind somewhere else. We are watching TV or reading a book or are involved in a business discussion while eating. The food becomes secondary, the tasks at hand primary. The meal gets over quickly and we often overeat. This is because the senses are not involved. Consequently, the satiety centre in the brain does not get activated.

Food is meant to be nourishment, not just for our bodies, but also for our minds. So a lot of importance should be accorded to not just what we eat, but also how we eat. All our senses and our attention ought to be on the plate of food while we eat. Concentrate on the variety of colours, hues and textures on your plate. Savour each morsel and then see the difference it makes to your eating. Concentrated efforts while eating leads to a blissful state and this is the essence of meditative eating.

ANTI-STRESS FOODS TIPS

What you eat or drink can in some way affect your mind. It can either calm you down or agitate you. There are a large number of anti-stress diets that claim to promote a soothing effect on the individual. Basically they aim at raising the serotonin levels or the feel-good chemical levels in the brain, which would elevate your mood and help reduce anxiety levels.

As stress increases the cellular activity, the body requires more nutrients. So these diets are high in their nutritional content. Stress also disturbs the smooth functioning of the digestive tract which again can deplete nutrition from the cell renewal process. Anti-stress diets try and provide the body with nutritional content in adequate amounts without tipping the delicate balance of the physiological process.

Anti-stress diets give credence to the following :

Do not Over-eat
Darshana Lathigra, a London-based dietician and lifestyle coach warns, "If you eat as if there is no tomorrow, there really may not be one". This is one of the basic tenets of anti-stress diets. Over-eating or food bingeing could be a potent stressor apart from creating obesity related diseases, Excessive eating can cause stomach distension, regurgitation and abdominal discomfort leading to stress. Hence an optimal intake is advised.

Do not Starve
Avoiding meals for long hours can lead to acid formation and irritation of the digestive organs. One is putting oneself in line for gastroenteritis, peptic ulcers and problems of flatulence and acidity. This is advised against by those on an anti-stress diet. Eating on a two-hourly basis is strongly advised. Eating every two to four hours helps to maintain your metabolism. By eating more often your glucose and insulin levels are kept in balance. Three to five small, but, wholesome meals a day is in fact recommended.

CHAPTER 13 : MEDITATIVE EATING

Stay Hydrated
Lots of water is important to keep us well hydrated and to help counteract stress by circulating nutrients. Water makes up approximately 60 to 70 per cent of the human body by weight, so all of us need to stay hydrated to keep our bodies running smoothly. Dehydration itself can cause headaches, fatigue and lethargy and can compound stress. So drinking at least 8 glasses of water everyday is advisable. Apart from water, juices and soups are also recommended as are fruits with high water content.

Just Eat While Eating
Avoid distractions, arguments and other activities like watching television or reading or working on the laptop during meals.

Relaxed Eating
Try to rest and relax before and after eating, even if just for a minute or two. It will help to take 10-15 minutes, time out around meals. Listening to relaxing music also helps.

Avoid Coffee
Drinking four or five cups of coffee in a day can cause changes in the blood pressure and produce stress hormone levels similar to those produced in chronic stress. Coffee is addictive, dehydrating and takes a long time to get flushed out of the system.

Soups and Salads
These are especially recommended in huge amounts as they have the potential to nourish us well without creating great demands on our body and digestion. Our energy level and productivity may rise with eating such foods that are refreshing and keep the nutritional content intact.

Anti-stress Nutrition
Green veggies, complex carbs, non shell variety of seafood cooked with low fat and spice content will help. It is best to avoid red meat,

shell fish and foods which are spicy and deep fried, to remain low stressed. Cigarettes and alcohol are prohibited. Moderate amount of dark chocolates can be taken as they are supposed to be a stress busters.

> Meditative Eating is the art of enjoying food with all the senses. Eating with awareness adds many more value to food apart from the taste.

CHAPTER 14

Visualization, in your Personal Theatre

It is said that things happen twice, first in the mind and then in reality. This concept was popularized by the great golfer Jack Nicklaus. He says that he has never hit a shot, not even in practice, without having a very sharp picture of it in his head. In his mind, he would first construct the swing, the ball trajectory and the place he wanted the ball to land. Only when he had a clear image of what he wanted, he would proceed with the shot.

Many sportsmen, industrialists and inventors have succeeded because they had a vision, a sharply etched dream. Think of yourself as a winner and the battle is half won. Think of yourself as thin and there is a high chance that you will lose weight.

Arnold Schwarzenegger, the famous Hollywood star says "The mind is the limit. As long as the mind can envision the fact that you can do something, you can do it, as long as you really believe in it 100 per cent."

So there are better chances of achieving your goal if you know what exactly you want. In fact, a lot of stress is created if the goal is not clear. There is bound to be vagueness, confusion, hesitation and an incomplete attempt at execution. Once the goal is established, you can plunge headlong into the task.

Creative Visualization is one of the ways in

> Nothing happens unless first we dream.
> *Carl Sandburg*

which you can make a complete picture of your goal in the mind. Your mind's eye visualizes and stores well-defined pictures of the future. Meditating on this picture may actually make your dream a reality. **Creative Visualization** in one sense is an improvement on 'the power of positive thinking' which extols you to be positive in your aspirations and it will pay dividends.

Apart from its role in helping achieve one's goal, Creative Visualization is a very popular mode of relaxation. Visualization or imagery is considered a very potent form of meditation, with proven stress-busting powers. Visualization is the art of activating a personal theatre in our mind. It is a theatre, where you can revisit the past, venture into the future and go on virtual vacations.

Our mind is like a mansion with many, many rooms. Many of these rooms are unused. They are in the ruins, gathering dust and cobwebs. These rooms like the music room, art gallery, dance studio, meditation chamber and the writer's nook are seldom used. These rooms are situated in the right side of the brain and our busy schedules leave us with very little time to go into these rooms.

Most of us tend to gather all our thoughts in a small room in the left side of the brain. This room gets crowded. Day to day mundane activities like paying bills, appointments, etc. reside in this room. I am not undermining the value of this room. This room is our lifeline; it is our air, food and water. However, it is required that we get out of this room once in a while. We need to cross over and visit the room on the right side. There is a lot of fun stored on the right side.

The mansion stands for our brain, and the rooms are the two sides of our brain. The left brain is primarily responsible for understanding language, speaking and writing. The receptor centres here stand for logical thinking, memory, analytical thinking etc. The left brain helps us remember names, telephone numbers, anniversaries and keeps an account of the money in the bank account.

The right brain thinks in pictures, sounds and feelings. Even if it forgets an anniversary it has a detailed memory of the way the eyes had met that first time! The right brain stands for creative thinking. Lateral thinking is aided by receptors of the right brain.

CHAPTER 14 : VISUALIZATION, IN YOUR PERSONAL THEATRE

The left brain analyzes, tear things apart, while the right brain synthesizes, putting pieces together. The left brain can remember all the words of a song, while the right would write a new song. The left is a logical thinker, while the right is more attuned to intuitions and emotions. The left is most concerned with the outer world of culture, agreements, business and time, while the right is more concerned with the inner world of dreams, aspirations and emotions.

I have a passion for the creative forms of expression and therefore crossover to the right part of the brain frequently. The entire process is akin to sitting in a personal theatre where I am both the audience and the enactor. I indulge in my theatre very often to refresh, so that I can take on the more mundane things of life.

HOW TO ACTIVATE YOUR PERSONAL THEATRE

While most of us can use imagery successfully, it needs a fair amount of commitment to get it right. Also, it is affected by one's patience and persistence. It's quite like learning to whistle or swim or ride a bicycle. First, you decide to do it, then you need to learn to do it and finally, get doing to actually doing it. You need to put in the time, effort and discipline to be able to indulge in imagery.

Imagery and visualization needs a lot of practice. Here are some simple steps to aid in visualization:

Relax: To create imagery successfully, it is necessary to relax. Assume a comfortable position. Unless you are using imagery to induce sleep, it is better to be seated. Use a chair with a backrest. Sit back on the chair so that your buttocks touch the backrest and your spine is supported. Take a few deep breaths. Ensure that your belly moves with every breath you take. Establish a slow breathing rhythm. Close your eyes and get ready to activate your personal theatre.

Select the Topic: The crucial step in the imagery process is to decide the topic for visualization. That keeps us focused and the details get sharpened. For example, if you visualize yourself on the beach, then you have to first create a beach scene in your mind. Let me show you how to do it right.

Imagine yourself standing at a gate opening to the beach. A narrow path leads from the gate to the beach. The path, which takes you to the sand, is paved with green shrubbery. The sand on the beach is pristine silver, virgin and sloping gently to the water. The sea is blue and you can see waves lashing on the silver sand. You can hear the roar of the sea and can feel the tide coming.

You can now enter the scene as an audience or an actor. Creative Visualization as a process involves setting of goals for the future, and being an audience helps. Processes that involve relaxation like taking off on a vacation to an exotic location can very well have you as an actor, playing the central role. In Creative Visualization or imagery a number of characters and situations can be brought into the frame. If you are planning for the future then you can position the people in your life like your spouse, children, parents, colleagues or friends as part of the visual frame.

Now start by visualizing yourself on a beach. Start walking on the beach. Feel the breeze on your face, in your hair. Feel your feet sinking softly in the sand, leaving beautiful footprints. Smell the clean, fresh air... Breathe deeply.

Pick up a little pace, and stride along with energy and vigour. Notice the tall palms swaying in the wind; watch the leaves in different shades of green. See the blue sky with an occasional cloud moving slowly with the wind. Meet your friend from school on the beach. You have not met him for years. Hug him. Sit him down and talk about the fun you had in school. Ask him about his family and you tell about yours. Visualize the rain. Feel the rain drops on your cheeks. The rain picks up and there is a steady shower. You try to run for cover but there is nothing nearby. You decide to get wet; enjoy getting drenched. Visualize all of this in your senses. Get involved totally in your dreams.

It is essential to visualize a happy ending. So, be sure to make the ending positive. There will be situations where you may land up with stray thoughts. Just as it is with other forms of meditation, you

CHAPTER 14 : VISUALIZATION, IN YOUR PERSONAL THEATRE

should gently brush away the thought and come back to visualization or imagery. As you finish your walk on the beach, you return to your cottage. Your family is waiting for breakfast. You introduce your school friend to your family and all of you sit by the pool and enjoy a hearty breakfast. Happy ending!

HOW DOES VISUALIZATION WORK FOR YOU?

Creative Visualization gives your subconscious mind a clear picture of what you want to accomplish. The pictures you create are stored in the subconscious mind, which drive you towards your goal. Just as you use imagery for relaxation, Creative Visualization helps you project your dreams, hopes and aspirations in the theatre of your mind.

If super fitness is your goal, start with your gym bag. You see yourself folding the clothes and putting them in your monographed gym bag. You walk down to the gym. The 5-minute walk to the gym serves as a good warm-up. You see yourself in the gym beginning your workout with stretches. One of your friends greets you and compliments you on your flexibility. You thank him.

Creative Visualization, of the future, works better if viewed as a third person. It gives you a chance to see yourself in the frame. You can see your shape, posture and movements. You can give yourself the desired shape in your movie. You can see yourself assume correct posture during your exercises. This remains in your subconscious mind and will help you with correct posture when you are actually exercising. While visualizing, you may get overlapping pictures or a negative thought or may even strike a blank. In this case, breathe deeply and bring your mind back to the scene gently. You could bring yourself back in the picture, the gym shoes you are wearing, the vibrant colors of your shirt, your muscles showing their new found shape...you will be back in business.

After stretching you do some cardio exercise on the treadmill. You visualize yourself picking speed and striding comfortably at 10 km per hour. Your heart monitor tells you that you are well in your training zone. You are sweating and breathing deeply, enjoying yourself thoroughly. After your cardio exercise you are now planning a 12 station circuit weight training session. You approach the leg press machine, adjust the weights and start pushing. You can feel your quadriceps working hard to press the weight you have selected. Your gym trainer is admiring your dedication and drive. You thank him and proceed with the second station.

After your weight training, you cool down and go for a shower. You feel the water spray on your body. Oh! what a pleasant sensation. After your shower you go for the fitness assessment room. Your weight is 75 kg and your fat content is 12 per cent. The gym trainer who is assessing you says that you deserve an award for your achievement. Your movie ends with 'A happy ending'!

VISUALIZATION: APPLICATION TO LIFE EVENTS

The most important application of Creative Visualization is perhaps the setting of a clear-cut goal. Knowing what you intend to get is half the battle won. Creative Visualization is a self-help technique that uses your imagination to manifest what you want in life, and creates a clear image of the goal. Constantly meditating on this image, and continuous feeding of this image many a times turns it into a reality. This is because it helps you remove or bypass any internal blockages or negative thinking within yourself especially in the subconscious mind that may be hindering your progress towards the chosen goal. Many good leaders are called 'visionaries' and most often than not they have been found to indulge in Creative Visualization. They see possibilities, dream of those possibilities turning into realities and plan every detail meticulously in their minds. So, when they actually get down to working on their plan, it turns out to be flawless, as the glitches would have been worked out during the visualization phase itself.

Some form of visualization is used by athletes everyday. Visualization has been recommended by experts such as Steven Covey and Dale Carnegie as a method to achieve peak performance in individuals. Athletes use visualization to enhance their performance, sometimes without realizing it. A fast bowler in cricket visualizes his run-up, delivery stride, and then pictures his ball beat

CHAPTER 14 : VISUALIZATION, IN YOUR PERSONAL THEATRE

the batsman and send the stumps flying. A golfer visualizes his swing, club hitting the ball straight and high right in the middle of the fairway. A tennis player may run a mental film of his serve which crashes into the wall as an ace! All this spurs the individual to liken his action to his dream.

Visualization may be good for creating a harmonious interpersonal relationship, especially when they are stress inducing. Sometimes even if you have the intention of apologizing to your spouse or child, it does not happen. There are a lot of mental blockages or inhibitions, which come between thought and action. Creative Visualization can be helpful here. You realize that you were very rude to your child the previous day. You want to rectify the matter. Visualize yourself taking your child for a walk or a drive. You buy him an ice-cream, and chat about things in his school. After the ice-cream has been eaten and relished, you tell the child that you are sorry for what you said yesterday. Visualize the expression on your child's face. You hug the child, ask him if you are forgiven, and continue with the walk or drive. A lot of disputes can be solved through dialogue or communication. By visualizing the dialogue a rehearsal is conducted, the mind is cleared of any blockages or inhibitions and the ice is broken.

Positive thought and constructive imagery can help in healing the body. Just as negative thinking and stress can lead to disease, visualization of a happy ending can favourably alter a physical ailment. Research shows that conditions including depression, impotence, allergies and asthma can be helped with visualization. Imagery can also be used to stimulate our immune systems. It is not an alternative to modern medicine, but can be used as a good adjunct or a complementary mode of therapy.

With imagery we can successfully block haphazard thoughts and streamline the mind. By taking mini vacations we can relax and feel refreshed. To enrich our visualization process and aid in detailing, it would help to take frequent real vacations and fill our mind with beautiful pictures. These pictures, already stored in our memory bank, can be brought back to life during the practice of imagery.

As we saw earlier, visualization is the domain of the right brain, the seat of creativity. Hence, as a pure extension of logic, visualization and creativity go hand in hand. A creative person would have indulged in it at some point of his life. Also, your creative potentials will get a boost with such kind of visualization.

Finally, this process really works for people suffering from lack of sleep. Imagery is particularly useful on a day when you are agitated and your mind is full of stressful thoughts. I use my favourite script of playing golf on a familiar golf course. I visualize myself slowing down the swing, slowing down the walk, breathing deeply, hitting the next shot, sinking, putting and proceeding to the next hole. I do not remember going beyond the third hole. Slowly but surely, sleep sets in. This not only helps in sleeping, but also diffuses the mind and turns it towards a more positive thought.

Visualisation is a wonderful medium, only if one believes in it and uses it in the way it is described above. Psychologists and therapists all over the world encourage disturbed and stressed-out individuals to indulge in some amount of visualization. This provides them with certain amount of positivism that is immensely important for their rejuvenation, revitalization and growth.

Baba Calm Dev is a product of my Creative Visualization. You can interpret this as a statutory warning, before embarking on Creative Visualization!

> Creative Visualization is the art of dreaming the end by creating an image of what you want in the future. The Personal Theatre is activated and the goal can be visualized in picture form. Imagery is also a powerful tool to accomplish relaxation and thwart stress.

Positive Affirmations

CHAPTER 15

"I am the greatest," said Muhammad Ali. He made this famous statement much before he became a legend and soon enough, greatness did follow him.

"I am the greatest" remains one of the most effective affirmations in history. Ali said it to himself, and to the world, because he believed that he would make unparalleled boxing history. Ali had a goal in mind, and with it had the technique, strength, talent and above all had belief in himself. He had made an Affirmation.

Affirmations are auto-suggestions or motivational self-talk aimed to focus on goals and build confidence. The aim of affirmation is to help the individual think in a positive way about oneself. You can overcome the barriers that stand in between you and the person you have always aspired to be.

How are affirmations helpful in stress management? Positive statements are very helpful in stress management. Stress creates and magnifies negative thoughts, which in turn creates more stress. A vicious cycle develops. Positive affirmations are a great tool to re-programme your subconscious mind and turn it away from negative thinking to positive ones. When you keep repeating positive outcomes, you start believing in them and they become part of you. In doing so, they lower stress levels. When you make an affirmation you make a promise to yourself in

> Saying is believing.
> *Baba Calm Dev*

a way and show faith in your abilities. So, affirmations are reaffirming and reassuring and ease out self-doubt.

Positive affirmations create a high level of confidence. Many actions in life are based on confidence. Whether it is answering an oral exam, facing an interview, speaking in public or hitting a good golf shot, confidence is vital. On the other hand, anxiety and nervousness are the impediments in way of good performance. While entering the exam hall a simple affirmation like "I am calm and relaxed" or "I am well prepared" can work wonders. This kind of positive self-talk acts like a mantra and helps to give one's best.

Affirmations help sportsmen, musicians and other performing artists to bring out their best. A mention of the word 'affirmation' brings to mind my good friend and fellow golfer Ajit Parmar. Though he condescends to play with us amateurs, he dresses, walks, thinks, visualizes and behaves like a professional. He is usually full of affirmations which imply that he is the best among us and in the end this is what is usually proved. Most of the games are won by him. What Ajit rides on is positive affirmation.

Performance-related anxiety does not spare any sportsperson, whether you are playing the US Open Golf Championship or a Sunday bet match with your friends. If a golfer is nervous, anxiety does not let him complete his golf swing smoothly. An amateur looks up to see where the ball is heading, and the swing is not completed correctly. Even a professional golfer makes mistakes under pressure, ending up hitting a bad shot. A positive affirmation can help by beating back negative thoughts and bringing in positive ones. The person gets charged up and feels encouraged with the thought that he can be the best. This confidence he gains after positive affirmation; something that lingers on long after the game is over.

So, positive affirmations create confidence, which influences action, usually of the positive and successful kind.

Apart from being used with great success in performance enhancement and stress relief, positive affirmations have a huge role in the medical world. Positive affirmations and positive

CHAPTER 15 : POSITIVE AFFIRMATIONS

thinking techniques can help develop a powerful and positive attitude towards life, which is an essential element in gaining and maintaining good health.

Positive affirmations can be helpful while recovering from an injury or recuperating after surgery. It is also useful in treating people suffering and trying to cope with a loss.

How to use positive affirmation to ease away your pain? Consider your injury and pain as something that is healing and going away. Speak to yourself positively every day about your ability to cope with and recover from your injury. Positive self-talk like "I am healing" or "I am feeling better" can actually favourably alter the recovery process. When it comes to healing, positive affirmations work best in conjunction with visualization and deep breathing techniques.

Positive affirmations can help you overcome addictions and vices. I say this from experience. I was a smoker in college and many attempts to give up smoking had proved futile. The day I came to know that Rashmi, my wife, was pregnant; I decided to quit smoking once and for all. I had no right to subject the unborn child to noxious fumes. This time I was not to fail in my 'butt kicking' venture. At a party I announced to myself and all around, "I have given up smoking" and chucked the cigarette packet in the bin. Unknowingly, I had a made an affirmation. This affirmation had a great effect on me. I have never smoked after that day. The public declaration complemented the affirmation. I was not going to lose face in front of my friends, being caught with a cigarette. Repeating the mantra "I have given up smoking" ensured that I did not hold a cigarette ever again.

Positive affirmations can improve human bonding. If you repeat "I love my wife" it can help reinforce your vows. The affirmation "I forgive you" can help you forget and forgive, and bury the hatchet in many relationships. Positive auto-suggestions can help you look at relationships with a much broader and mature outlook and bring harmony in life. Trivial matters often lead to irreversible differences. Positive affirmations which look at the foundation of a relationship will help you bypass triviality and strengthen the bond. Positive affirmations can help you quash ego and usher in happiness and contentment.

Positive affirmation can help you create universal goodness. **Aham Brahmasmi** literally translates to 'I am God'. No, it is not a sentence credited to an egoistic orthopaedic surgeon. It is one of the oldest affirmations, often repeated in the *Upanishads*. In this ecstatic statement of enlightenment, 'I' does not refer to the self or the individual or our outer form, but to the essence of the soul which is ever inseparable from Brahma or the Supreme Being.

Aham Brahmasmi suggests: My soul is linked to God. Khalil Gibran has expressed a similar concept when he says 'I am in the heart of God'. Repeating such a positive affirmation may not cause instant enlightenment but it can usher in feelings of goodness and empathy towards all around us. It also is a positive step towards global oneness.

HOW TO MAKE POSITIVE AFFIRMATIONS
Identify the Goal
Affirmations can begin with the end in mind. What is it that you want? If you came across Aladdin's magic lamp, what would you ask the Genie for? Is it more happiness, peace, better relationships, more money, a healthier lifestyle or something else? It would be better to write them down and ruminate and brainstorm till the goals become crystal clear. After you have established what it is you want, think about the actions and the attitude needed to reach that goal.

Construct a Statement
Depending on the goal, you can make a positive statement which will help you proceed in that direction. Affirmations when repeated often start to reside in the subconscious mind. They help you to get focused and energize and channelize your energies towards the goal. They reinforce your self-worth and make you feel confident for the task ahead. With positive affirmations you can instruct your

CHAPTER 15 : POSITIVE AFFIRMATIONS

body and mind to act in the way you want. If you are a singer and want to give a great performance you could make a statement 'I am the best and I rock'. Believe in the affirmation and you will be the best.

Make it Personal
The affirmation will be more effective if it is pertaining to your personal goal, rather than a generalized statement. 'I am a good putter' will work better for a golfer than a nonspecific statement like 'I can accomplish anything'. A specific personalized affirmation keeps your goal in focus and pushes you towards it.

Be Positive
Positive is different from 'not negative'. 'I am a good putter' is better than 'I am not a bad putter'. This means saying what I want to be reinforced and not what I want to avoid. Sometimes the human mind doesn't register the negative, and it just hears the word "bad" which is what needs to be avoided.

Speak in the Present Tense
Affirmations made in present tense work better than those in the future tense. 'I am a good putter' is more effective than 'I want to be a good putter'. The mind registers the present tense and believes that the your putting is already good. An affirmation like "I am happy" suggests that happiness is already present and proves more relaxing than a statement 'I want to be happy'.

Visualization Helps
Affirmations which can be pictured and played in the personal theatre become more dynamic with added dimensions of colour and sound. These affirmations can be used in conjunction with creative visualization, especially for healing purposes. As you say, 'I am feeling better' you can visualize the pain being herded out by the imaginary elves.

Make a Mantra of the Affirmation

The effect of the affirmation can be multiplied by repeating it often. Like a mantra you could repeat the affirmation several times in a day. The mantra could be chanted aloud making it even more effective because you hear it too. With modern mobile phones and other portable devices providing voice recording facility, you could record your affirmation, which can be played back at will. My personal favourite affirmation is 'I am Calm'. And it works.

Writing down Affirmations

The written word can be of great value in reinforcing the affirmations. I know of a friend who writes his affirmations in his diary everyday. As he goes through his appointments and other day to day work, the affirmations remain in his perspective. Another good method is to write your affirmations on chits of paper which can be stuck to refrigerators or cupboards.

BEYOND AFFIRMATION: SELF-HYPNOSIS

Self-hypnosis is a practical and effective technique for relaxing deeply. It is an affirmation taken to another level. Here the person is drawn into a trance-like state, to a level where he is open to suggestions. Self-hypnosis happens when he is open to suggestions by himself. It is an extremely useful tool that can be used for everything; from simple relaxation to pain management to increasing one's chances of success.

I have seen a presentation where tooth extractions and minor surgical procedures were performed without anaesthesia and under the influence of hypnotic suggestion. In fact, it is often used by psychoanalysts to heal people of their anxieties and pain.

Relax

For self-hypnosis you need to find a quiet place, with little distraction. A comfortable position is desired. An easy chair with a good lumbar support works well. If you recline, there is the possibility of falling asleep. Hypnosis works best at the point where

CHAPTER 15 : POSITIVE AFFIRMATIONS

the person is in a trance like state but is open to suggestions. It works at the level of the subconscious and unconscious.

Give a Goal to your Session

Self-hypnosis requires a goal to operate. If you are a singer who is having trouble touching high notes, then the goal should be to create suggestions that you are comfortable with high notes. Make a positive statement to that effect. The statement could be, "I can sing high notes easily."

The Technique

Start with deep but easy abdominal breathing. Imagine yourself breathing in calmness and exhaling all the tension. Once you feel completely relaxed, use the affirmations you have prepared. Now imagine that you are in a beautiful music chamber, with beautiful musical instruments lined up. Listen to the soothing strains of the violin as you sit down to soak in the atmosphere. Keep visualizing and hearing the various instruments come to life in the orchestra. Continue the deep breathing. Many can go into an altered state at this point. You feel totally relaxed and at ease, as if in a dream world.

At this point when you are in a zone of total relaxation, feeling far away, in some distant world, you can start the auto-suggestion. You can now start repeating "I can sing high notes easily". After about 20 repetitions of the affirmative statement, you may choose to visualize the affirmation and see yourself singing a high note. Your voice is steady, the note is sustained and there is thunderous applause. You are singing the high note easily. This is a sure way to cement the affirmation into your subconscious mind.

Self-hypnosis is easy to do, inexpensive and the results are lasting. Self-hypnosis helps you to relax your body, lets stress hormones subside, and distracts your mind from unpleasant thoughts. There are no potential negative side effects, and it can give multiple benefits at the same time. All you need is some free time, a quiet place, comfortable clothing, a desire, a relaxed open mind and a clear idea of what you want.

Self-hypnosis has helped many people reduce stress, quit smoking, manage pain and improve performance. Musicians, sportspersons, motivational speakers and other achievers have acknowledged the benefit of self-hypnosis. Try it, you will definitely enjoy.

> Affirmations are positive motivational auto-suggestions, which work like mantras as they abolish self-doubt and add to your self-confidence. Affirmations in conjunction with visualization can help your dreams come true.

Laughter

CHAPTER 16

He who laughs... lasts.

Laughter is the best medicine!

Laughter is internal jogging!

Laugh lines lengthen lifelines!

"A day without laughter is a day wasted" – Charlie Chaplin.

Laughter has now entered mainstream medicinal interventions in a big way. There are laughter clinics and laughter clubs that have mushroomed all over the globe aiming to elevate the mood and alleviate misery. In the USA there is an association which deals with therapeutic aspects of humour. In fact, I have visited a centre doing research work in therapeutic laughter called Hasya Yoga Kendra in Mumbai. There are some composers writing laughter music!

> Chicken soup for the soul for me, and don't forget to add some laughing stock.
> *Baba Calm Dev*

WHY LAUGH?

We seem to have underestimated the value of laughter. It, in fact, has many proven benefits to the mind and body. So let's start laughing and make this life richer.

INTRINSIC BENEFITS OF LAUGHTER

Laughter has intrinsic and extrinsic benefits. Intrinsic benefits include a better mind and body. Mood elevation while laughing causes the release of endorphins in the brain. You really feel better after watching that funny movie or TV serial; you feel relaxed. It is due to the presence of endorphins.

Benefits of laughter include compulsory deep respiration. Hearty laughter involves effective expiration of gases followed by deep inspiration, a good exercise for your lungs and diaphragm.

Laughter is a wonderful stress-reducer and antidote to upsetting events. It is clinically proven to be effective in combating stress, although the exact mechanism is not known. Experts say a good laugh relaxes tense muscles, speeds more oxygen into your system and lowers blood pressure. Read a funny book or call a friend and chuckle for a few minutes. It even helps to force a laugh once in a while. You'll find your stress melting away almost instantly.

Americans were attracted to humour from the stories of Norman Cousins, who had successfully overcome cancer by watching comedy shows on television. Benefits to the immune system too have been documented. Regular hearty laughter ensures higher levels of immunoglobulins, which increase your immunity.

Several philosophers have recommended laughter as a form of meditation. When you laugh you forget the world and live in the moment completely. There is no worry of the past or worries about the future. You are in the present, enjoying yourself, completely lost to the world. Laughter can be a transcendental experience.

Researchers are gathering more and more evidence that laughter can be used as a form of therapy to alleviate pain in terminal illness. Where highly potent analgesics fail, laughter has shown good results. Laughter has shown arrest and reversal of several chronic diseases of the psycho-somatic variety.

The future looks good for the development of laughter as a form of alternate medicine with holistic dimensions. Besides, laughter has not as yet killed anyone, nor has it shown to produce any side effects. So laugh your way to a stress-free life.

EXTRINSIC BENEFITS OF LAUGHTER

Laughter has several extrinsic benefits, which essentially means that by laughing you can pass on some benefit to others. This is the concept of passive laughing. Laughter is infectious and can change the mood of a gathering. It can improve the working environment

CHAPTER 16 : LAUGHTER

in an office, ease tension and enhance creativity. A sense of humour is a rare quality in a person and probably the most sought after.

WHY HAVE WE STOPPED LAUGHING?

Babies laugh a hundred times a day and adults only a few times. Children communicate by crying and laughing, the fundamental human languages irrespective of race or creed. However, during the process of growth and development, one loses these basic emotions due to a process of education and conditioning. Children are often subject to a tirade of advice like:

- Wipe that silly grin off your face!
- What's so funny?
- Don't laugh like a jackass!
- Learn to be serious.
- Have you gone mad? Stop it.

Soon we get conditioned to suppress laughter and one day it becomes difficult to laugh heartily.

HOW HIGH IS YOUR LQ OR LAUGHTER QUOTIENT?

Many of us boast of a high IQ or an intelligence quotient but have we looked into our laughter quotient? Laughter quotient tells us the ease with which we can laugh. Higher the LQ, easier it is to laugh at the smallest of things. Lucky are those people with high LQ.

We had a very pleasant person called Raghu in our medical college. He was very popular as he had a high LQ. Jokes were graded according to the intensity with which he laughed. Raghu was called Jokometer Raghu and we would get immediate feedback of our pranks and jokes from his laugh. If your joke failed to elicit a laugh out of Raghu you were pits in the humour department.

Once a professor said to Raghu: "Stop laughing. Doctors should be more serious." Raghu replied solemnly: "Sir, It would be beneficial to us doctors if patients were more serious."

WHERE DO I FIND LAUGHTER?

If you develop the attitude then there is humour everywhere. Life is full of puns and satires, paradoxes and slapsticks, funny sounds and sights. All one needs to do is look around and see the funny side of life. I come across such instances all the time.

One day, when my son Nishad was about 4 years old, we were to go out for dinner, after my clinic hours. He and his mother were to pick me up from the clinic. He came into the clinic, while his mother waited in the car. I was waiting for the last patient to arrive, and told Nishad that we could leave for dinner only after I was done with the last patient. Nishad started playing in the waiting room.

The patient was a little delayed but he finally arrived. When he entered my chamber he had a strange expression on his face. He asked me if everything was OK. He also enquired about my practice. I told him that things could not be better, and thanked him for his concern. Then he told me the reason for his concern. As soon as he entered the waiting room, a child saw him and started jumping with joy, yelling "Patient has come; patient has come; now we can go have dinner"!!!

Therefore to stay fit, healthy and happy, we need to look for humour in day to day situations. Try laughing at the chaos and unpredictability in life. We could develop a cartoonist's perspective. Dr. R. K. Laxman, India's most creative cartoonist deserves accolades for getting that smile on the faces of millions of readers in spite of the terrible news headlines staring at them.

If you can do something to help the situation, do it. If you cannot...just laugh your worries away.

> Finding humour in a situation and laughing your heart out can be truly therapeutic. Laughter, the most natural non-verbal expression of joy, keeps you rooted to the moment just as it makes you breathe deeply. It floods your body with the elixirs of happiness. A true stress buster.

CHAPTER 17

Put Your Worries to Sleep

It is a lazy monsoon afternoon in Goa. There is a mild drizzle. The sea is choppy and a gentle breeze is blowing. From my cottage I can see the palms swaying in a steady rhythm. But I am in danger of being deported. I have broken a major rule of the Goans. I am writing this chapter while all of Goa is indulging in *sosegad*. Instead of poring onto my laptop, I should be curled in bed enjoying the midday sleep like the rest of Goa.

Sosegad, is one term that best exemplifies the lifestyle of the people of Goa. It goes hand in hand with the other Goan mantras of music, dance, food and feni. *sosegad* complements the Goan philosophy of wholeheartedly celebrating every moment of life.

Sosegad is derived from the Portuguese root word *socegad* which means quiet. Like the dance and music, *Sosegad* is a fond remnant of the Portuguese influence on Goa. *Sosegad* or siesta is part of the Goans' daily routine when they rest in the afternoon, come what may. Activity in Goa comes to a quiet halt in the afternoon with the shops closed between 1 and 4 pm. It is *sosegad* or siesta time.

The word siesta also originates from the Portuguese word *sesta*, the traditional daily midday sleep of Southern Portugal. This way of life gradually spread to Spain and later to the Latin American countries. In these countries,

> You can wake up to the idea that a catnap can bulldoze all worries.
> *Baba Calm Dev*

the heat can be oppressive and unbearable in the early afternoon. The heat probably ushered the tradition of taking a midday break, to literally 'chill out' in the comfort of one's own home. Besides the climate, in many countries it is common to have the largest meal of the day in the afternoon. Thus, a siesta may also be a natural sequel to this large meal.

Today, the term siesta refers to a short nap for about 15 to 30 minutes, usually taken after lunch. They are more of a light rest and are often interchangebly used with other words like power nap, catnap, snooze, doze, kip or winks.

As a doctor practising in Mumbai, siesta is not alien to me. Most doctors in private practice work in two sessions. The mornings are utilized for surgeries and hospital rounds and the evenings for seeing patients in the clinic. The time in between is siesta time, after a sumptuous meal at home.

Siesta is colloquially known as "Boporiya", derived from the Gujarati word for afternoon. Boporiyas can have different connotations, where one need not sleep alone nor is it mandatory to be in one's own home!

Siestas are also seen at orthopaedic conferences, during the afternoon session, where the speaker's oratory is applauded by sonorous snores. The audience at these conferences hog a heavy lunch, which induces postprandial dip in blood glucose levels. This caused by the body's normal insulin response to a heavy meal, producing drowsiness. The speaker's voice acts like a lullaby; soon we have loud sound sleepers.

HOW LONG SHOULD THE SIESTA BE?

When you sleep under normal circumstances, your brain enters several different stages of sleep, which are delta, theta, alpha, beta, and gamma sleep waves. You drift from one stage of sleep to another — from light sleep to deeper sleep to REM sleep to wakefulness and so on. Delta and theta sleep, also known as Sleep I and Sleep II stages, are light stages of sleep. So, the key to napping is to not fall into the deeper stages of sleep.

CHAPTER 17 : PUT YOUR WORRIES TO SLEEP

As far as the siesta is concerned, many experts advise you to keep the nap short and sweet, between 15 and 30 minutes. Sleeping longer gets you into deeper stages of sleep, from which it is difficult to awaken. Deep sleep in the afternoon can make it more difficult for you to fall asleep at night.

However, some other studies have shown that an hour's slumber has many more restorative effects than a 30-minute nap. The mental faculties are better rested and made more ready for the challenges later in the day. There is a thin line between waking up in a groggy state and opening your eyes feeling refreshed. It is often not the deep sleep but the interruption of your sleep cycle that makes you groggy. You have to understand your own sleep cycle and decide the length of the siesta.

As the opinions differ on the ideal length of sleep, you could let your schedule make the decision. If you have only 15 minutes to spare, take them! But if you could carve out an hour from your work, you may as well complete a whole sleep cycle. If you only have 5 minutes to spare, just close your eyes and relax. Even if you do not sleep, a brief rest has the benefit of reducing stress and helping you relax. A few minutes of eye-shut can give you more energy for your day ahead.

HEALTH BENEFITS OF SIESTA
Siesta for a Healthier Heart
The siesta can be used to combat stress and it improves the functioning of the heart. A recent study conducted on 23,681 Greek men and women found strong evidence in support of siesta. It was found that individuals who took a midday nap for 30 minutes or more, at least three times a week were 37 per cent less likely to die from diseases associated with the heart. Mortality rates also came down by 34 per cent. Among working men who were into the habit of taking a siesta, a 64 per cent reduced risk of heart disease and death was found. The study clearly supported the theory that all other variables remaining constant, a midday rest or sleep contributed to a lowered risk of heart disease.

Siesta for Improved Performance and Efficiency

This is self-explanatory and almost everybody knows that the body repairs and feels rejuvenated after a short nap. Siesta invariably gives mind the time to rest without lapsing into deep sleep and inactivity. So, the mind wakes up feeling energized and this is manifested in the performance levels and efficiency. In one study, subjects were asked to perform a visual task of identifying diagrams on a computer screen. It was found that their scores on the task worsened over the course of four daily practice sessions. Allowing some subjects a 30-minute nap after the second session prevented any further deterioration in their scores, while a 1-hour nap actually boosted performance in the third and fourth sessions.

Therefore, short naps do improve performance whether it is in the field of academics, research, sports, business and any other endeavour. Many busy executives who are deficient on regular night time sleep, make time for short naps during the day. Steve Fossett made his record 67-hour flight around-the-world alone in his jet and stayed energized with power naps. When Lance Armstrong was training for the Tour-de-France bicycle race, naps were an important part of his routine. In Iraq, U.S. Marines are instructed to take a power nap before going on patrol. Students whose schedules are interspersed with short naps are able to do much better than those who study at a stretch. Short naps aid in memory retention and improve recall.

Rest for Neck and Back

The siesta or afternoon nap can give your back and neck a much deserved rest. The computer has become a way of work and life for many. The posture adopted at work through the day can cause physical and mental stress. The neck and back are the most affected. A short rest, ideally in the horizontal position will relax the muscles and provide great relief to the spine.

CHAPTER 17 : PUT YOUR WORRIES TO SLEEP

NAPPING TIPS
Do not Feel Guilty
Tell yourself that you are not being lazy by napping. Make an affirmation that napping makes you more productive and more alert. Knowing that you are not napping at the expense of your work will make the nap even better. Know this for a fact that napping will improve your performance level.

Select a Particular Time
Try to nap just after lunch; human circadian rhythms or biorhythms make early afternoons a more likely time to fall into a productive nap zone.

Say No to Coffee
Avoid consuming large quantities of caffeine as well as foods that are heavy in fat and sugar, since these meddle with a person's ability to fall asleep. Instead, switch to foods high in calcium and protein since they are known to have qualities that promote sleep.

Nap in a Quiet Place
Find a clean, quiet place where external disturbances are either cut off or minimized. Wear an eyeshade or draw the curtains. Darkness stimulates melatonin, the sleep-inducing hormone.

Take Note of your Posture
It is very important to assume good posture while napping. Thirty minutes of sleeping at the desk with a crooked neck can be disastrous. A stiff neck is the last thing that you would want. If a couch is available, go for it. Lie down in a horizontal position and enjoy the nap. If your chair is the only option, it would be wise to procure a neck support pillow, like the ones given on long flights.

Deep Breathing
A few deep breaths and a visualization exercise will help you nap quicker.

Music

Soft background instrumental music is very conducive to napping. However, this is only for those who can sleep with music in the background. Switch it off if it distracts you. Also do not play rhythmic music since it makes falling asleep difficult.

Ideal Temperature

Remember that body temperature drops when you fall asleep. Raise the room temperature or use a blanket to aid sleep.

Set Alarm

Once you are relaxed and in position to fall asleep, set your alarm for the desired duration so that a power nap or a siesta remains just so...a siesta.

The *sosegad* or siesta time is not over as yet. I can surely squeeze in a nap. Zzzzz......

> A short midday siesta can recharge your batteries and energize you to enjoy the tasks ahead. Apart from performance enhancement, a siesta has proven health benefits, especially on the heart.

CHAPTER 18

Massage

Massage is something that is not a novelty in India. In fact, we Indians have been exposed to it since our birth. New born babies are given an oil massage every day before their bath so as to promote circulation and promote strength and vitality in those little limbs. New mothers, post delivery are also given massages to restore their muscular strength and improve blood circulation. Haircut sessions are incomplete without a short complimentary head massage or *maalish* thrown in by the barber. There is a famous Hindi film song, which proclaims that an oil massage to the head can be a panacea to all the troubles in life. Of course, the therapeutic value of the Ayurvedic massage from Kerala is world famous. Also popular are the Oriental massages especially those that originate in Thailand. These days face massages are also gaining ground and modern parlours as well as the *maalishwalas* co-exist because of the plentiful opportunities in this field.

> I am really touched when I am given a massage.
> *Baba Calm Dev*

WHAT IS A MASSAGE?

A massage is defined as a structured touch, applied to the superficial or deep tissues, muscles, or connective tissues, by applying pressure on them through manual means. Such application may include friction, gliding, rocking, tapping, kneading or stretching. The practice of massage is designed to promote general relaxation, enhance circulation, improve joint movement, relieve stress and ease muscle tension, with an aim to promote a general sense of well-being.

A massage therapy would include a skilful manipulation of the hands over painful muscle areas and tissues so as to lessen pain, improve muscle tone and circulation and induce relaxation. Massages are often used to treat soft tissue ailments and supplementary aids such as alcohol, liniments, oils, antiseptics, powders, herbal preparations, creams or lotions, hot or cold packs are used to provide relief.

The human touch involved in massage, significantly adds to its therapeutic value. The medicinal value of human touch cannot be overemphasized. Physiotherapist Dr Richa Kavade says, "The doctor's touch conveys empathy, compassion, hope and understanding making touch in itself an important part of pain alleviation."

HISTORY OF MASSAGE

The concept of massage is not new and the power of touch in healing is a well documented theory. In fact, in India, massages have been used to arouse forms of dormant energy in the individual. For example, the use of a tantric massage to arouse Kundalini form of energy has been in practice since the ancient times. Similarly, documented evidence has been found in Chinese writings, dating back to 1400 BC mentioning the use of massage and burning herbs as a method of treating disease.

The history of therapeutic massage can be traced to the 5th century BC in Greece. Hippocrates, the father of modern medicine, said "A physician must be experienced in many things but assuredly also in rubbing." He advocated massage along with fresh air, good food, bath, music, rest, and visits to friends as the key to treating disease. Aesculapius, another 5th century BC healer in Greece, promoted massage in conjunction with herbs, diet, relaxation and hydrotherapy.

In the 6th century AD, the Japanese developed the art of Shiatsu massage to manipulate energy within the body. The word Shiatsu itself means applying pressure with the fingers.

CHAPTER 18 : MASSAGE

Sweden's Henrik Ling (1776-1839) is considered the father of modern Western massage. His 'Swedish Massage' spread from Sweden, over the course of the 19th century, into Europe and America. His system was based on a keen understanding of physiology and formalized a series of gymnastic movements along with massage techniques.

In 1895, a Society of Trained Masseuses was formed in Britain to increase the standard of training and in 1899, Sir William Bennet inaugurated a massage department at St. George's Hospital, London.

The amalgamation of massage into sports training schedules started at the 1924 Olympic Games in Paris. Paavo Nurmi from Finland brought a personal massage therapist to the running competition and won 5 gold medals. Nurmi claimed that his training programme included this special massage treatment.

The manual element in a massage has been somewhat excluded with the invention of the massage chair by David Palmer. This device aims at promoting total body relaxation and helps in stress release and relaxation. However, masseurs are still in demand and cost far less than the massage chair. In addition the chair takes up a lot of space and is not very aesthetic in nature. Hence, it has not really taken off and the massage parlours as well as the *maalishwalas* still hold forth over the market.

HOW DOES MASSAGE WORK

Massage works at two levels; at a central level it provides a feel-good factor, and at the tissue level it works on the muscles directly.

Our bodies and posture are held in balance by the muscular system. In order to stand still there are various muscles throughout the body constantly contracting and relaxing to maintain your posture. If one or more of your muscles become too tight or slack then your posture will be affected. If this is not corrected, over a period of time, you will have a permanent muscle imbalance and onset of degenerative disease.

Massage therapy comes in handy to correct muscle imbalance

and altered posture. The muscles which are too tight are relaxed and stretched, and the ones that are too slack are toned. If a joint is too tight causing stiffness then it is mobilized.

As an orthopaedic surgeon I recommend massage in several chronic back and neck conditions. Backaches and neck problems caused due to muscle tightness respond very well to massage therapy. Selecting a trained masseur is of utmost importance.

Massage is however never recommended in injuries. Whether it is a muscle pull or an injury due to a direct impact, massage has no role to play in the treatment. An injury needs to be iced and rested. A massage can aggravate an injury by creating more swelling and inflammation. Back problems like prolapsed inter-vertebral discs and spinal instabilities can be damaged further with massage.

TYPES OF MASSAGE

There are many types of massage. Some techniques are stimulating while others are relaxing. Some use the basis of modern anatomy and physiology, while others use traditional concepts like energy systems and *kundalini*. Some techniques claim to be highly therapeutic and curative while others highlight their feel good value. From the many techniques of massage described and practiced, one has to choose what is suitable, available, safe and enjoyable.

Ayurvedic Kerala Massage

The Ayurvedic massage system with the fragrant oils and baths have shown to possess power to heal as well as relax. Kerala, with its rich cultural heritage, has kept alive this ancient art of therapeutic healing and popularized it throughout the globe. In fact, tourism in Kerala heavily banks on these therapeutic massages. The Ayurveda has a holistic approach to healing, where diet, meditation, herbal preparations and massage sessions work in tandem to facilitate well being.

Swedish Massage

The most common type of modern massage in the Western world is

CHAPTER 18 : MASSAGE

the Swedish massage. Massage therapists use long smooth strokes, kneading, and circular movements on superficial layers of muscle using a lubricant such as a massage lotion or oil. Swedish massage therapy can be very gentle and relaxing.

Aromatherapy Massage

Aromatherapy massage is a massage therapy with the addition of one or more essential oils. These are used to address specific needs. One of the most common essential oils used in aromatherapy massage is lavender since it promotes relaxation. Oils of lemon; eucalyptus, rose, tea tree, etc. are also used. This form of massage is particularly suited to stress-related conditions.

Deep Tissue Massage

Deep Tissue massage targets the deeper layers of muscle and connective tissue. The massage therapist uses slower strokes or friction techniques across the grain of the muscle. Deep tissue massage is used for chronically tight or painful muscles, repetitive strain or postural problems. People often feel sore for a day or two after such a massage.

Shiatsu

Shiatsu is a form of Japanese bodywork that uses localized finger pressure in a rhythmic sequence on acupuncture meridians. Each point is held for 2 to 8 seconds to improve the flow of energy and help the body regain balance.

People are normally pleasantly surprised when they try Shiatsu for the first time. It is relaxing yet the pressure is firm, and there is usually no soreness afterwards.

Antenatal Massage

Antenatal or prenatal massage is becoming increasingly popular with expectant mothers. In the early days, such massages were given by untrained *dais* or midwives. However, these days massage therapists have taken their place. They are usually certified practitioners especially in the area of a pregnancy massage, who know the proper way to position and support the woman's body during the massage. They also modify techniques to suit the pregnant lady. The procedure is customized according to the needs of the woman. Pregnancy massage helps to reduce stress, decrease swelling, relieve aches and pains, and reduces anxiety and depression. The massage is customized to a woman's individual needs. However, care must be taken that the masseur is trained or else there could be complications.

Sports Massage
Sports massage is specifically designed for people involved in sports and other physical activities. But you don't have to be a professional athlete to have one. It is also used by people who are into exercising. The focus is on relaxation, making the body more supple, supine and strong. It also prevents injury and enhances performance. Sports massage uses a combination of techniques and the strokes are generally faster than in a Swedish massage. Before an event, stimulating manoeuvers are used and after the event the massage aims at relaxing the tired body.

BENEFITS OF MASSAGE
General Benefits of Massage Therapy
There is no doubt that massage makes anyone feel good and it is a pleasurable experience. Massage increases your body's self-awareness and sensitivity. Massage reduces your stress, tension and anxiety levels by working on the mind as well as the tissues.

Benefits your Muscular System
Massage increases the blood supply and nutrition to the muscles and helps your muscles recover more quickly from exertion and fatigue. Massage relaxes your muscles effectively reducing spasms, tension and cramping. Massage helps to prevent muscular atrophy or wasting from injury or paralysis.

Benefits your Skeletal Systems
Massage improves the circulation and nutrition of the joints and helps increase the range of joint movements through releasing tight muscles and tendons.

Benefits your Circulatory Systems
Massage increases the strength and nutritional content of the tissues by increasing the blood circulation to the tissues. This is due to the mechanical actions which produces a dilation of the blood vessels. By improving venous drainage, massage enhances the elimination of the waste products of your metabolism. Due to the relaxation response, massage has the overall effect of lowering your blood pressure and reduces pulse rate.

Benefits your Nervous System
Massage can have a sedative, stimulating and invigorating effect on the nervous system depending on the type and length of treatment given. Massage through touch and the right kind of pressure stimulates the proprioceptive receptors of the skin and underlying tissue making the person relaxed and calm under the effects of the skilful hands of the masseur.

Total Body Relaxation
A good massage can promote an overall sense of well being. As nerve impulse conductors move the stimulus from one receptor to another throughout your body, each part will begin to relax and bask in a delightful sensation of comfort and rest. Massage suppresses the release of stress hormones and increases the levels of seratonin, the feel-good hormone.

Enhanced Relationship
"Massage helps you stay in touch" says Baba Calm Dev. The power of touch can work wonders in your interpersonal life. Exchanging a massage with your spouse can bridge gaps, build stronger bonds and make the relationship better rooted and grounded. Most

relationship therapists emphasize on the power of massages in couples who have distanced themselves from each other usually due to intense work pressures. They say that massages help develop a greater level of trust and collegiality especially when physical intimacy is involved.

Massage ensures golf for me on Sundays. My wife Rashmi, has a Sunday noon date with her masseuse or *maalishwali*. Her *maalishwali* has soft hands and a silken touch, and Rashmi has got quite addicted to it. So come what may, she wants the exclusive rights to our bedroom during the massage hour. My presence in the house has sometimes caused a hindrance in the well-oiled mechanics of her massage. Golf is suggested to me and with feigned reluctance I drag my feet to the course!

Massage pampers the body by providing human touch as well as improving the blood circulation in the tissues. The tension in the muscles just vanishes with massage. Very few stress busters can match the instant relaxation provided by massage.

Calm Sutra of Sex

CHAPTER 19

Sex and stress have an intricate relationship. On the one hand sex is recommended as a stress-buster, on the other, sex itself has been a cause of lot of stress. Unfulfilled desires, fantasies, under performance, deviations, infidelity, fear of pregnancy, fear of sexually transmitted disease, have all contributed to great levels of stress. While the sex addict can give stress as one more excuse to have sex, the under performer can blame stress for his lack of desire. Sex hormones and stress hormones are often seen to be inversely proportional to each other. If one is high, it is more likely that the other will be low.

As we have seen earlier, stress can lead to diminished sexual desire and an inability to achieve orgasm in both men and women. In fact, it can lead to erectile dysfunction in men and sometimes even temporary impotency. Part of the stress response involves the release of brain chemicals that constrict the smooth muscles of the penis and its arteries. This constriction reduces the blood flow into the penis and increases the blood flow out of the penis, which can prevent erection. Hence stress is highly avoidable for those who want to lead a happy and healthy sexual life.

Even though we all agree that highly stressed persons could easily de-stress with sex, sex isn't always included as a top stress management technique; although in my opinion it ought to be. It is hugely physically

> When the seven year itch is over, you better start from scratch.
> *Baba Calm Dev*

and emotionally satisfying and hence it can help people perform better at their work place and be more positive in their dealings with the world. Let us see how a healthy sex life can help manage stress.

SEX IS AN EFFECTIVE STRESS BUSTER

Apart from effectively diverting your mind away from your worries, sex provides many stress management and health benefits.

Sex as an Exercise

Sex, if nothing else, is an invigorating exercise. One can pleasurably burn some 200 calories. This is about the same as running 15 minutes on a treadmill or playing a spirited game of squash. The pulse rate, in a person aroused, rises from about 70 beats per minute to 150, the same as that of an athlete putting forth a serious effort. Muscular contractions during intercourse work the pelvis, thighs, buttocks, arms, neck and thorax. If some of the Kama Sutra poses were to be followed, one could easily improve flexibility and muscle co-ordination. Sex also boosts production of testosterone, which leads to stronger bones and muscles.

Sex as Meditation

Sex makes a person totally immersed in his moment. In fact, sex as a communion with God has been the premise of many ancient rituals; sex was indeed looked upon as a spiritual act. However, things have changed in the present times with power games being enacted and manifested through the act of sex. Still, sex therapists do emphasize on the value of a good session in bed. The anticipation, the act and the post sex relaxation, all ensure that you are at the moment with the person you want to be, in a moment of total commitment. All the troubles seem to dissipate after the act of physical intimacy since it lends a touch of security, love and faith to the relationship. In fact, post 9/11, sexual togetherness rose among Americans. It is this oneness of the mind and the body that lends a meditative angle to the entire exercise of sex. Sex performed mindfully, with full awareness, is a form of dynamic meditation, popularized by Osho for which he had to face a lot of flak from purists and the moral police.

Deep Breathing
The excitement and the physical activity associated with sex can produce deep abdominal breathing. It induces a rhythmic breathing that is done in unison and this relaxes the body, provides more oxygen to the blood, builds up energy and reduces the stress. All the health benefits that accrue out of breathing are further enhanced by the pleasurable act of sex.

Sense of Touch
The act of sex and foreplay involves physical touch. Studies show that touch, which is a vital component of massage can be a great stress reliever. In fact, touch promotes emotional health. Research also shows that babies who are not physically touched enough by way of cuddling, lifting etc. grow up to be emotionally deprived. Sometimes, in extreme cases they fail to thrive. Touch continues to play a pivotal role in adulthood and in the very act of acquiring physical intimacy, by way of hugging and kissing, makes touch a very important factor in promoting health and vitality.

Sex, Endorphins and Pain Relief
Sexual activity releases endorphins and other feel-good hormones. Endorphins are released due to multiple reasons in sex. The physical workout, the deep breathing, the massage component involved, the positions... all contribute in the release of the wonderful elixir endorphin. Immediately before orgasm, levels of the hormone oxytocin surge to five times their normal level. This also helps release endorphins. In women, sex also prompts production of estrogen, which can reduce the pain of PMS.

Sex and Immunity
Wilkes University in Pennsylvania says individuals who have sex once or twice a week show 30% higher levels of the antibody called

immunoglobulin A, which is known to boost immunity. Sex consequently reduces the chances of colds, flu and other ailments caused by lower immunity.

Sex Improves Self-worth
Sex brings with it a feeling of being wanted. Sex is an extension of non verbal praise or appreciation of the physical form of the partner and an expression of being attracted. Sex, thus makes you feel better about yourself and adds loads to your self-esteem and self-worth.

STRESS MANAGEMENT FOR BETTER SEX
Sex can be a great stress reliever, with the physical and emotional release, bonding, and release of endorphins. On the other hand, stress can actually prevent us from being 'in the mood'. Excessive stress can dampen the libido, reducing the drive, frequency and intensity of sex. Stress can drive you to a life of involuntary celibacy. The following stress relieving measures can help you rejuvenate your sexual drive and performance.

Sexy Foods
You are what you eat, goes the saying, and it holds true even in the matter of sex. The type of food you ingest can energize you or make you sluggish. The food you eat can either calm you down or make you stressed. A healthy, balanced diet with plenty of vegetables, protein and whole foods can actually reduce your stress level, increase your energy, and help your body look and feel better. This will go a long way towards getting you in the mood for sex. Though some sexologists recommend shellfish and other sex stimulants, the role of these aphrodisiacal foods is often questioned. On the other hand a quiet candle light romantic dinner will probably usher in an arousal, no matter what is eaten.

Exercise
There is no doubt that exercise can be a big turn-on. A tired person

CHAPTER 19 : CALM SUTRA OF SEX

can actually be energized with exercise and driven to romance. A romantic walk or a gym session with your partner can be a stimulant to love making. Studies have shown that certain exercises like weight training can stimulate sex hormones which have a positive effect on your libido. Exercise makes you happier with your body, makes you more attractive and adds to your sex appeal. A fit person is fit to try more positions as prescribed in the Kama Sutra and add variety to his sexual life.

Sleep your Way Through Stress
Adequate sleep is essential to thwart stress. Sleep deprivation can cause stress and wreak your sex life. Sound sleep at night and a power nap or siesta can help you have all the energy for a good romp in bed.

Calm Sutra for Kama Sutra
With a regular practice of one or more relaxation techniques described in Calm Sutra, you can reduce the stress and tension you feel in your body and mind. Having some of the tension gone, you'll feel freer to express yourself sexually.

Laugh Together
A sense of humour connects two beings as nothing can. If you laugh together there is chance you will want the company of the other. This is a great way of bringing on the mood for sex. Laughter being a great stress buster can work wonders in making a couple come together.

Get Closer Emotionally
Stress affected by change can throw your sex life out of gear. Moving house or having a baby may have you preoccupied elsewhere, with little attention towards sex. This is the time for emotional bonding. Get connected emotionally, do things for each other, take joy in the most mundane of things and build up your connection with each other at the level of the mind. The body will follow.

Take a Break
Best sex is had on holidays. A relaxed mind, far away from the day to day worries, will ensure a good stimulus for sex. A boat ride in a lake, followed by a walk to the hotel, a glass of wine, a journey into the past and you have a perfect setting for love. Music, aromatherapy, and a soothing environment can all help set the tone for relaxation and romance. A little preparation can yield some great results!

Spice it up with Variety
Variety can go a long way in providing a deeper connection. You might want to start differently by massaging your partner. Massage is known to have aphrodisiacal properties. Bring in variety in your moves, in the areas that you use. Be more receptive to the desires of your partner. Provide love, respect and above all a security blanket for your partner and this would be the right way to experience the magic of sex.

FURTHER READING:
Sex is Not a Four Letter Word by Dr Sudhakar Krishnamurti.

Apart from providing mutual pleasure and happiness, sex enhances self-worth and esteem. A healthy sex life is a powerful tool for stress management.

CHAPTER 20

Music

Music means different things to different people. For most music is a form of entertainment, something to listen to and relax. For others it is something they can dance to, while for some others it is an expression of their love and devotion to God. Music is poetry, an expression of human emotions, and therefore, a beautiful manifestation of all things good in life.

People take to music in various emotions. In happiness as well as in sorrow, music has immense power to absorb and heal. People use music to relax and feel leisurely. However, people also use the rhythm and the beats of music while exercising, dancing, painting, working at home and in office, driving etc. Many others use music to help them meditate. The music in this situation is more monotonous and soft.

In the past, great musicians like Tansen and Baiju Bawra used to control the elements of nature with their powerful and melodious music. However, things have changed now. Music and its power to heal has been recognized and it is increasingly being used as a therapy. In fact, music therapy is a popular mode of therapy that is used to calm down agitated minds, erase painful memories, heal the person and make him a complete whole. With the vast outreach of music and the universal language that it speaks, music is

> Music beats the blues, soundly.
> *Baba Calm Dev*

used to promote peace, goodwill and global oneness.

Calm Sutra celebrates music.

HOW HAS MUSIC WORKED FOR ME?

For me music has been and continues to be a vital part of life. Music brings me unparalleled joy as I listen to it or sing or play the keyboards. It takes me into another world and I can spend hours constructively listening to music.

Music helps me relax. Music makes me dance, makes my exercise more enjoyable. Through music I continue to make many friends.

Music brings me memories and I can travel back in time as some old songs are played. Music has helped me visit the right wing of my brain, dabble in poetry and try and write some tunes. Music for me has metamorphosed from a hobby and source of entertainment, into a medium for meditation and inward bliss.

WHAT IS MUSIC?

Music is defined as organized sound. For sound to be termed music, it should be pleasant and have melody, harmony and rhythm, fused into a synchronised whole. The word music comes from the Greek word 'mousikê' and also from the Latin word 'musica'. Music was probably inspired from mousa, the Greek word for muse.

Though music is considered an art form, there is a lot of science which goes into music; it is the science of acoustic, which involves the key elements of pitch, timbre, texture, tone and rhythm. Frequencies of sound are arranged in specific sequence so as to produce a sound that is pleasing to the ears. Therefore, in an orchestra or a concert, a conductor's full score is a chart or a graph, which indicates frequencies, intensities, volume changes, melody, and harmony etc. put together in a sequence. This sequence has to be adhered to within a time frame. In a sense it is like mathematics, precise and accurate and this is what produces music that remains etched in the listener's memory long after the instruments have been put to rest. Speaking about the intricacies of music, noted mathematician, Pythagoras asserted in the fifth century BC that,

CHAPTER 20 : MUSIC

"There is geometry in the humming of the strings. There is music in the spacing of the spheres."

Apart from its scientific and mathematical dimensions, music has a human and emotional facet, which attracts people towards it. Music has the capacity to reach your heart and tug at your feelings; it transcends the barriers of language, time, caste, creed, colour, geographical location and touches the feelings and emotions of its listeners. It is a universal language of thoughts and emotions.

MUSIC AND STRESS

Music does wonders to alleviate stress and is the most preferred option for many. This has been proved in a study where people were asked to name any activity they preferred to indulge in to beat stress. There were 24 activities given as choices. It was found that almost 64 per cent preferred listening to music as a way to relax. It was closely followed by television with 53 per cent opting it as a first choice. Indulging in sex, taking a bath or going to a therapist had very few takers. This shows the immense power of music in healing stressed minds.

Music is a significant mood-changer and reliever of stress, working on many levels at once. Music is known to reduce heartbeat rate and increase body temperature, which itself indicates the onset of relaxation. Combining music with relaxation therapy has shown to be more effective than doing relaxation therapy alone.

Experts have suggested that it is the rhythm of music, essentially the beat of the score that has a calming effect on us. Developmental psychologists have pointed out that babies in their mother's womb were close to the heart beat of their mother. Hence, when they are nestled close to their mother's heart while sleeping or suckling, they immediately calm down and drift off to sleep. This soothing feeling is replicated in various kinds of music that we experience as adults, perhaps associating it with the safe, relaxing and protective environment provided by our mothers. Research has shown that rhythmic music stimulates the brain and ultimately causes brainwaves to resonate in time with the rhythm. Faster beats are known to encourage more alert and concentrated thinking. Slow beats encourage slow brainwaves that are associated with hypnotic or meditative states.

However, there are others who feel that it is the melody that has a calming effect on the individual. The melody creates vibrations in the body, which can trigger energy systems to drive away stress. This theory is based on the principle of resonance, which means that the precise harmony contained in a particular musical piece resonates inside the human body. The sound is picked up by the receptors in the ears and transmitted to the brain and from the brain the vibrations pass on to various organs. The melody in music stimulates certain biological processes; the sensory organs relieve certain sensations attached to the music and this helps in the abatement of stress.

There may be a debate on whether it is the rhythm in the music or it is the melody, which soothes us. But there are no two thoughts that music soothes. For further proof you need to meet my friend, Dr. Anil Tibrewala. Apart from being a leading cosmetic surgeon he is a fantastic singer deeply rooted in music. Stress just eludes him.

MUSIC AND MOODS

Music does create a mood, whether it is to do with romance or fear or fun, music can enhance the mood. As kids, when my cousin Veda and I used to watch a horror movie, she used to instinctively shut her ears. She would keep her eyes on the screen but shut out the audio inputs. She used to say that it was the background music which made the movie scarier. Elimination of music playing during the chilling sequence, made the scene far less frightening. Many years and many movies later I learnt that the visual media depended on music to create the magic of a scene.

In fact, restaurants, malls, movie halls, shopping arcades, play schools etc. have all understood the power of music and taken recourse to it to create the right mood and ambience. Films are designed to convey a certain mood, feeling and sometimes even the

CHAPTER 20 : MUSIC

audience it is targeted at. Is it a fun film for a young audience? Chances are that it will have some fresh, hip sounds that are more rhythm based. A movie that deals with the underworld will never have bubblegum music. So, composers have a challenging job to create music keeping a definitive purpose in mind.

Music usually sets the mood at restaurants and shopping centres. At a take-away, the music will be more catchy and rhythmic and will be engineered to keep you on your toes. In a proper sit down restaurant, the music will be slow, soft, soothing and will probably be in line with the décor. It will be designed to whet your appetite.

With the advent of mobile phones and caller tunes, people go out of their way to select specific music to greet you. When you are calling someone or are kept on hold, the caller tune creates an impression of the person or the organization you are calling. Recently when I tried calling an estate broker, I was greeted by a melodious 'mantra'. I enjoyed being kept on hold and the music emanated a good vibe instantly. I had begun to like him even before meeting him. Thus music definitely creates a proper befitting mood.

The ragas in Indian classical music are mood based. A raga is a system of sequencing musical notes to create a melody. Each raga is associated with a definite mood or sentiment that nature arouses in human beings. The ancient musicologists were particularly interested in the effects of musical notes on moods. They studied the effect of sequenced musical notes in enhancing human behaviour. They recognized that music had the power to make you feel happy, sad, refreshed, energized and even supremely motivated. War songs charged up the soldiers and patriotic songs infused a feeling of pride for one's own country. A lot of research has gone into this aspect of music and its power to evoke a myriad emotions.

Indian classical music has a number of ragas, each studded differently with the seven *swars* or notes. These ragas also have a time assigned to them to create the right effect. It is believed that only in this specified period, the raga appears to be at the height of its melodic beauty and majestic splendour. There are some ragas for the early hours of the mornings like *Bhairav*; others like *Yaman* appeal in the evenings, yet others like *Malkauns* spread their fragrance only during the midnight hour. This connection of time of the day or night, with the raga is based on daily cycle of changes that occur in our own body and mind.

I have experienced ragas creating magic on my moods, even as they mesmerize me with their melody. We were invited to an early morning concert of the great Hindustani classical vocalist, Pandit Jasraj. The Gateway of India in Mumbai provided the perfect backdrop for the concert, which began well before sunrise. Panditji sang devotional compositions in morning ragas. As Panditji's voice warmed up, we saw Mumbai being illuminated by the first rays of the sun. The melody of the morning ragas created a divine atmosphere and words cannot describe the effect they had on us.

MUSIC THERAPY

Clinical studies have shown documentary evidence of health benefits from music. The benefit of music on living organisms was demonstrated on plants in an experimental study. It was found that plants which were subject to soft, soothing music grew lush green as compared to those subject to harsh, loud music. The plants also grew towards the source of the music that they liked. This amply proved the power of music in rejuvenation.

Music therapy has been used effectively to manage pain and improve mood and mobility in conditions like degenerative joint disease. Subjects with osteoarthritis reported less arthritic pain when music was played as compared to a control group who simply sat quietly. Many studies have shown the incredible effects that music has on chronic pain. People suffering from back pain, fibromyalgia, chronic fatigue syndrome, and pain from injuries; all benefit from using music. Physical therapy is much more effective when combined with music. And burn victims experience much less pain when soothing music is played during their treatment.

People undergoing surgery have been shown to require lesser dose of the anaesthetic, awaken from anaesthesia more quickly and with fewer side effects, when 'healing' music was played before,

CHAPTER 20 : MUSIC

during and after the surgical procedure. Music has effectively reduced the need of pain relievers and sedatives in the post operative period after major surgery.

It is well known that music relieves anxiety and eases depression. Individuals suffering from depression need less medication and have more success in psychotherapy when music is added to their course of treatment. Grief, loneliness, and even anger can be managed much better when appropriate music is added to therapy.

Objective reduction of blood pressure has been documented with music therapy in patients with hypertension. Certain kinds of music have been found to lower heart rates, respiratory rates, blood pressure, and increase tranquil mood states. Music has the capacity to regulate heart and breathing rate and increase oxygen levels in the blood. For individuals with hypertension and related conditions, music can be included with other therapies to promote health.

Music has the power to enhance concentration and improve creativity. Music helps you remain in the moment as you immerse yourself in the world of melody and rhythm. The activity of making music or the act of creating melodious sound is itself an incredibly powerful healing tool. Physical, mental and emotional health takes an upward swing when one makes music! It need not be of the level of a professional standard. Anything that is soulful and emerges straight from the heart touches the chord. It could be singing, humming, whistling, beating a drum, playing an instrument or actually composing a tune, anything can help. When music is made out of love, it heals.

In spite of growing evidence that music heals, it is yet to be accepted as a branch of mainstream medicine.

GETTING STARTED

To get the best out of music one needs to develop an 'ear' for music, a taste so to say. The ear allows you to enjoy various facets like the pitch, harmony, rhythm patterns and other nuances of music. The ear is the one which makes the music. To become a good singer or an instrumentalist, it is necessary to first develop the aptitude and

CALM SUTRA : THE ART OF RELAXATION

the attitude for it. Train and sharpen your senses, in this case the ear, towards each individual note, and you will know whether you have hit the right note. Some people are born with this talent and some can develop it with training. The training is best provided by a music teacher or a *guru*. A good teacher can lead you to the threshold of the musical world, from where you can step in, explore and discover the hidden musician in you.

I was lucky to be born in a musical family. Almost all my relatives were trained in some form of music or another. Indian classical music was the focal point of almost all discussions and popular Hindi film songs were dissected to find out which raga they were based on. I grew up in this healthy musical atmosphere and developed a taste for music. However, I took to it seriously under Rinku Das Gupta, my music teacher or *guru*, who trained me in the finer nuances of music. It helped that I already knew the basics of music. With a strong interest and aptitude I took to music like a fish takes to water. Even today I enjoy my music and after a long, hard day, it helps me definitely unwind and de-stress. I keep the music in me alive.

My wife Rashmi is to be blamed for creating a singer out of me. For a long time I enjoyed being a harmonium player or keyboardist at parties and social occasions. But Rashmi was sick of waiting till the fag end of a musical evening, as the accompanist would be the last to leave. She decided to make a singer out of me, with more flexi timings. She had no idea what she would be in for! Rinku Dasguptaji, my music teacher, was summoned and my vocal training started. Now she has to stay back even longer. Even after the musicians have long gone, I succumb to mild persuasion to carry on the singing into the night.

KARAOKE: HELPS IN TRAINING

Music lovers could not have asked for a better invention. Karaoke is a system where the music track of a song plays in the background and you can sing along. These tracks are available on compact discs or tapes, which you play on a music system, plug in a microphone and start singing. The inventors have excelled by creating a karaoke machine where computer chips are loaded onto a portable microphone system. This device can be attached to any TV set and you are ready to croon. Not only are you provided with the background music, the words appear on the TV screen, which give you good vocal cues. The karaoke machine is good for practising singing, for small performances and can even be the life of a party. The karaoke system has an inbuilt recording device, which lets you play back your performance and even gives you a score.

My father, who took to singing when he was 69 years old, swears by the concept of karaoke. His day is not complete without his stint at either practicing or recording his songs with karaoke tracks in the background. The addiction to karaoke is pretty strong and it often threatens to eat into his TV watching time. His 70th birthday was celebrated with a private release of an album with retro Hindi songs sung by him.

I strongly recommend karaoke for music lovers. It may help you release the singer trapped inside you. It is a good device, which keeps you rooted in the moment and in the beautiful company of melody. It gives you practice, training and opens up a beautiful world of music, poetry and imagination.

MEDITATING TO MUSIC

I find music the easiest and most effective medium to achieve a meditative state. The vibrating resonance of sound has the power to create total awareness of the present in a creative and leisurely way. Meditation can be achieved by listening to music, performing music or dancing to music.

Meditative listening is an art. I recommend Indian classical music, since it helps in setting the right mood. It is soft, soothing and has a rich quality. Be careful while choosing the raga as a wrong raga could spoil the mood. Devotional songs work just as well to set the mood. Beautiful music is available on compact discs, which can be loaded on your laptop or any other portable music-listening device and enjoyed through the day.

It is necessary to assume a good posture for effective listening. An arm chair with good back support is required. Take a few long, deep breaths and then switch on the music. Shut your eyes and begin a musical journey. Headphones are better suited for meditative listening as your attention is less likely to be diverted.

Listen and absorb the music with an open mind. Make no judgements. Also, do not allow yourself to be disturbed while at it. Treat this time as pious to gain maximum benefits. Let your ears absorb all the melody and let the music touch your entire body. It will ultimately reach your heart.

Music performed on the stage or elsewhere is a potent form of meditation and is recognized by all who indulge in it. Whether it is classical music, rock or pop; whether it is singing, playing an instrument or mixing music on the console, music can be meditative. When the mind is completely in tune with the melody and in time with the beat, you cannot be elsewhere. You are one with the music that you are hearing and this is the time when nothing else really matters.

Personally, I have meditative tracks of the *tanpura* in my car, on my laptop and cell phone. The monotonous drone keeps me in a meditative state whenever I choose to be. The Calm Sutra *Swar* meditation helps me achieve a meditative and blissful state and takes away my pain and worries of the day.

> Music not only provides entertainment, it is a true mood elevator. In the company of music you can dance and exercise or simply let melody and rhythm transport you to spiritual bliss.

CHAPTER 21

Dance Away your Blues

Dance as a celebratory form has existed since time immemorial. Ancient tribes danced in celebration, in preparation for war, to usher in the elements or to drive away ghosts. Even today we dance to express our happiness. Dance is the most exhilarating language which uses the body to communicate and release emotions, pent up or otherwise. This makes dance very therapeutic since it is a valve, which lets you release a lot of stress.

Dance energizes the body and soothes the mind. It involves the use of the entire body and is therefore a fairly energetic form of exercise in most cases. Aerobics is a modern form of exercise, which amalgamates some form of dance to work out regimes and is immensely popular. Fitness levels can be augmented with dance, whatever the type you choose to indulge in and is a fun way to enhance health and happiness.

Dance and music go hand in hand and one is incomplete without the other. In fact, dance does help you appreciate music and its nuances of rhythm better. Many successful musicians have taken lessons in dance to imbibe better rhythm into their music.

Dance, especially to soft music, can be very romantic and extremely sensual. Dancing with your partner can also strengthen bonds and create a level of intimacy that can be very warm and mood alleviating.

Dance is a form of dynamic meditation and

> Put on your dancing shoes, and dance away your blues...
> *Cliff Richards*

many dance forms are known to transport the dancer into a spiritual zone. This is especially true about Indian dances. Indian dances whether classical like Kathak, Bharat Natyam, Kuchipudi, Odissi or a more modern ballet form, have their genesis in devotion and surrender to the Almighty. This makes dance a complete form of meditation, especially dynamic meditation. Those who believe in this core concept get lost and immersed in their devotion to God while they dance. I have seen the transcendental effects of dance in the eyes of the Indian diva, Hema Malini. She often gets lost in the love and devotion of Lord Krishna, as she performs on stage and when she performs as Durga, she conveys the immense strength and spirit that is the embodiment of the goddess.

I am fortunate to have been associated with dance from a young age. As a child I attended a unique institution called the Vyayamshala. In many Indian languages, *Vyayam* means 'to exercise' and *shala* means 'school'. Apart from exercise, the school also taught us a dance form called Lezim.

Lezim is a vigorous group dance where the dancers perform choreographed movements set to different rhythm patterns. The foot movements are intricate and strenuous with a lot of lunges, squats and spins thrown in. The hand movements are performed by using a wooden staff chained to percussive cymbals. The mini cymbals create a sound in sync with the beat of the drums. The Lezim dance not only helped me in enhancing my fitness, it ingrained a sense of rhythm at an early age. Later, in college, it was great fun performing the Punjabi Bhangda as well as joining in the festive Daandiya Raas.

Recently, my wife Rashmi and I enrolled for dance lessons in traditional ballroom dancing. It was a great experience learning the Waltz and the Foxtrot. During the course, I realized that such dances were not just about grace and fluidity of movement, rather it was a great way of burning calories and staying fit. Since then, as a medical practitioner, I put a lot of emphasis on dance as a way to maintain and improve fitness levels.

HEALTH BENEFITS OF DANCE

"There are short-cuts to happiness, and dancing is one of them", says Vicki Baum.

There is no dispute that dance has many health benefits. In fact dance is now being used as a form of therapy. Dance is a recognized fitness modality with great effect on all the major systems and organs in the body, including the mind.

Dance is a Stress-Buster

Dance ensures that you stay in the moment. A choreographed dance demands full concentration and involvement. The mind should be completely focused on the rhythm and the dance steps. This leaves little room for worrisome thoughts and soon you get immersed in the dance. Dance being closely linked to music, brings with it all the stress busting attributes associated with rhythm and melody.

Dance Improves Posture

Dance involves the entire body as also the mind. It involves body co-ordination and balance. It also improves the same. It improves muscle function and adds grace and fluidity to the body in day to day activities. Dance makes a person more aware of his body. This will help him to take corrective steps to make his posture better aligned. A dancer sits better, stands better and walks better as a result of practiSed body awareness. With dance ingrained in your system, life soon becomes a series of artistic movements; smooth and effortless. Life then becomes a poetry in motion!

Cardiovascular Fitness

When you dance vigorously, your muscles need more oxygen, and the circulatory system works hard to bring it to them. That's why your heart beats faster and you start to pant. Most dance forms improve cardiac function by giving the heart and lungs a great workout. Ballroom, Jazz, Bhangda etc, any of these dance forms can give the dancer a workout. Studies have shown that dance can favourably affect blood pressure and keep it under control by making the body go through a host of exercises and movements that are useful for the cardiovascular system, and most importantly provides an outlet for pent up emotions. All these help in reducing stress and associated disorders.

Fat Loss
Dance can be an effective and enjoyable way to lose fat and control weight. Studies show that belly dancing burns 250-300 calories per hour. More dynamic forms like the Bhangda could burn more than 800 calories in an hour.

Good for Bones and Joints
Dance is a weight bearing activity which improves bone quality. Dance can be helpful in preventing osteoporosis. Dance also encourages your joints to remain mobile and ensures better lubrication. Sedentary activities like sitting still all day at work and in front of the television in the evening can make lose your flexibility. Dance with all the foot and upper body movements can help the joints regain their flexibility.

Better Muscle Tone and Body Shape
Dance can be helpful in improving muscle tone and strength. Many dance forms have incorporated squats, lunges, jumps and twirls, which work out the muscles in the body. In certain forms a dancer is required to lift up his partner which if done in the right way builds and tones the arm and leg muscles. All these activities help in muscle building and toning.

PRECAUTIONS WHILE DANCING
There are various precautions that one needs to follow while indulging in dance so that one does not miss out on the enjoyment without causing harm to the body.

As a doctor, I have seen numerous dance-related injuries due to improper form and technique. Break-dance knees, salsa hips and other such nomenclatures may soon find a place in orthopaedic literature. Many of these injuries are due to overuse, poor fitness, improper pre-dance routine, unsuitable dance floor or faulty footwear.

Warm-up and Cool-down

A dance session needs to be preceded by a proper warm-up and a stretching session. Many dance forms come close to athletic activity and need the pre-dance routine to ready the body for the rigours of the main dance. The dance session must end with a cool-down session to gradually bring the body back to the baseline activity level.

Form and Technique

A good teacher is essential to ensure proper form and posture during dance. A faulty technique could put excessive strain on certain body parts and make them susceptible to injury.

Monitor Fitness Levels Before Indulging in Dance

Certain dance styles are vigorous and put excessive demands on the heart, lungs, muscles and joints. Those who are grossly overweight or with cardiac problems, hypertension or suffer from arthritic conditions should consult their physician before embarking on strenuous dance regimes. It would be worth starting with a walk or cycling programme to attain a basic fitness level. Also check with your doctor before you start on a dance regime.

Optimum Dance Floor

A dance floor should be conducive to movement. An uneven or slippery dance floor should be avoided, as it would lead to injury while dancing. Modern dance studios have excellent flooring designed for mobility and providing the right bounce from the surface. Do enquire if you do not know much about the flooring. A dance floor that is conducive to your dance is worth every minute of your time and inspection.

Footwear

Proper footwear is always prescribed so that the joints and muscles are not put to strain. Ballet and other Western forms of dancing require footwear and so the dancer must ensure that the footwear is not sub-standard. However, most Indian dances are performed barefeet and here there is precious little that one can do. In this case it is wiser to check the type of flooring and then start on the practice.

GET STARTED NOW

Dance has certain madness to it, a certain vibrancy of form, movement and even colour. It is visually appealing especially if one understands the fine distinction between art and vulgarity. Hence, dance as a release to stress is an extremely preferred option for therapists across the globe. Whatever be the motivation for putting on your dancing shoes, dance has a lot to offer in terms of stress reduction, weight reduction and pain reduction. It can work wonders for your social life too since it helps you to meet people. So, select your dance style, try and find a facility close by and swing your way to life that is full of beauty, grace and happiness.

> Dance energizes the body and soothes the mind. Dance is a valve, which lets you release a lot of stress. Dance is a fun way to enhance health and happiness.

CHAPTER 22

Exercise: A Potent Stress-Buster

Robert Maynard Hutchins says, "Whenever I feel like exercising, I lie down until the feeling passes."

This is one of the most popular sentiments related to exercise. Most people are aware of the benefits of exercise and the ill effects of not indulging in the same. Still, there are very few people who have an exercising regime. This is mostly because exercising calls for a disciplined and strict regime and most people feel a little stressed out at the thought of opting for a gruelling schedule. However, those who are passionate about health, fitness and workout highlight the benefits accruing out of exercising. Exercising gives them a feeling of confidence about their bodies which is manifested in the way they deal with the world.

The association between exercise and suffering probably goes deep into childhood and stays on in the subconscious till adulthood. Most of us as children have been punished for misbehaviour and asked to run a couple of rounds in the playground. The subconscious mind equates running with suffering. On the other hand, a good performance is often rewarded with a chocolate leading to the concept of reinforcers. Chocolate becomes a positive reinforcer while exercising becomes a negative one. We live

> There are bad days and there are days that I exercise.
> *Baba Calm Dev*

with these concepts as adults and find it difficult to break away from them.

People take to exercise because of the feeling of pleasure and confidence they get. They often feel lighter and fitter after they have exercised and this is what makes them come back to it again.

These days, a lot of young people are opting for a fitness regime in their pursuit for a better and toned body. The celebrity circus along with the media has been largely involved in creating the notion of fitness and beauty. Almost everybody wants to be like the media-created stars with toned, fit and slim bodies. Also, a lot of celebrities are launching their sports apparel line, equipment and videos making exercising a very preferred option for the younger generation.

HEALTH BENEFITS OF EXERCISE
Exercise Increases the Size of the Heart
With exercise, the heart muscles increase in size, and with it increases the cardiovascular fitness levels. The size of the heart increases and it strengthens in capacity. Thus, when a person is at rest the heart has to beat lesser number of times. It is like using a bucket to transport water instead of a glass. You would be making lesser trips with the bucket. A fit person with a lower resting heart rate would be conserving a lot of heart beats, and this could contribute to a longer life.

Cardiovascular fitness would not only add years to your life but add life to your years. The quality of life improves when the limits of physical endurance improve and you have abundant energy for your diurnal activities. Further, blood pressure, lung capacity and oxygen utilization by the blood are better maintained and unnecessary use of drugs to combat illnesses is reduced.

The changes in the musculoskeletal system are usually apparent and visible. The muscles when exercised develop a healthy tone and firmness, which adds shape to the body. The muscle cells actually grow in size and strength. Stronger and more flexible muscles adapt better with the aging process and make the body mechanically more efficient.

CHAPTER 22 : EXERCISE - A POTENT STRESS BUSTER

Better muscles and posture help in maintaining the integrity of structures like the back, neck and knees that have tendency to degenerate with age. The bones have shown to strengthen with exercise. Exercise improves the bone mass and reduces the incidence of osteoporosis. This is of great importance to females around menopausal age where bones tend to lose calcium and become weak.

Reduction of fat is one of the biggest gains of exercising. It reduces the Body Mass Index (BMI) and accelerates the metabolic rate. This helps in burning more calories. The fat levels drop from the waist and the hips leading to a fitter body. This is a fine incentive for most of us. Fat reduction has many health benefits, like the joints function better, the heart is not overworked, you get less tired and your posture and your figure or physique definitely improves.

Exercise and Sex

The sexual desires and performances both increase with fitness gained through exercise. As fitness improves, you look younger and are more confident It also makes you more desirable.

A healthier heart can tolerate exertion better, making sex less fatiguing and more enjoyable. Better flexibility enables you for more postures and variety. The frequency as well as the duration of sex improves with fitness. The feel of a warmer, stronger and shapely body is better than a cold, fat, atonic body. Thus fitness helps you both psychologically and physiologically towards sexual fulfillment.

Exercise and Money

Fitness and money seem to be directly proportional to one another. A fit person could earn more due to increased production capability, energy and drive. The mornings are pleasant and one looks forward to a day of good work. Persons undergoing fitness programmes are more committed about increased efficiency and performance. It keeps one more agile and focused, which helps in increased productivity. Often this leads to promotions, better opportunities and associated financial climbs. Exercise improves one's state of health and brings down the costs incurred in medical bills. For example, a diabetic with diet and exercise could save a lot of money on expensive anti-diabetic drugs. An exercise cycle will be far cheaper than going in for a bypass surgery.

Exercise and Sport

More fit a sportsman better the performance, is the basic principle of sports. This is why exercising is very important for a sportsperson. An athlete with a low fat ratio, superior powers of endurance, flexibility and strength has a great advantage over his less endowed adversaries. Better fitness is associated with lower incidence of sports injuries which in turn ensures more life to a sportperson's career. In fact, it is also associated with a better mental attitude and confidence, which contribute towards better performance. That sports greatly benefits from exercises is aptly summed up by my friend and avid golfer, Ajit Parmar. He says, "My golf scores were often bad due to tiredness creeping in towards the closing stages of the game. I then embarked on a scientific diet and exercise programme. Today I am able to concentrate better, I am less tired and even my golf swing seems to have improved, all thanks to fitness." The incidence of injuries reduces with improved fitness, at all levels of sport.

You are a winner when you exercise, both from inside and outside. The outer winner comes in the shape of a better looking you, who feels more confident, feels far more energetic and puts in a better performance in almost every sphere of life. It makes you fitter, healthier, full of beans and ready to take on new challenges.

The inner winner makes you know yourself better. This self-awareness would lead to increased self-esteem and consequently, a more positive you. This has been the topic of many research papers. In real life, I have been witness to many increased self-esteems arising from exercising zones. Exercising brings self-control, which helps when one tries to tackle stress and bring down the physical and mental turmoil to more tolerable levels.

If you don't know your worth, you are not worth knowing —
Baba Calm Dev

CHAPTER 22 : EXERCISE - A POTENT STRESS BUSTER

WHY IS EXERCISE A REAL STRESS-BUSTER?

When asked how they coped with stress, a large percentage of people indicated that they use exercise as their primary coping mechanism. This is a paradoxical situation since exercise produces a physiological response in the body almost identical to the one produced by stress and yet it is a potent stress-buster. Let us learn how?

During the stress response a huge number of biochemical reactions occur in the body. Neurotransmitters are activated, hormones are released, and nutrients are metabolized. During the fight/flight response, the cardiovascular system increases its functions and the gastrointestinal system slows down its operations in response to stress. These reactions are similar to that which were produced in prehistoric times when men needed to fight for survival and required these bursts of expend physical energy.

In modern times, most human stress is psychological in nature and the need to respond physically is not necessary. However the same levels of energy are needed to combat stress at the psychological level. The byproducts of the stress response like cortisol continue to circulate in the body and have the potential to create physical illness. Exercise depletes some of these resources in an acceptable way so that the individual does not fall ill. Regular exercise allows the body to maintain good metabolism or homeostasis and reduce the physical impact of stress.

Exercise increases the production of certain chemicals like endorphins. These endorphin levels have been shown to increase during physical activity of twenty minutes or more. Chemically, they are similar to opiate compounds like morphine and can provide an analgesic or pain relieving effect, as well as create a sense of euphoria. Athletes have actually described the feeling of a psychological boost after exercising and named it the runner's high. Several researchers have however questioned this theory for its lack of empirical evidence. The theory is unable to exactly measure chemical changes that occur on the other side of the blood-brain barrier.

Regardless of the understanding of the exact neuro-chemical reaction or other mechanisms that initiate changes in emotional status, this phenomenon does seem to exist. Research is under way to correctly identify factors. The positive mood states associated with frequent exercise are so palpable and significant that some therapists believe that exercising can be a more effective treatment for clinical depression, especially, if it is administered along with drugs and psychotherapy.

Exercise: An Outlet for Emotions

Exercise is a great outlet for pent up anger and hostility. A good whack to the golf ball or a series of punches to the punching bag can be a catharsis for negative energies and caustic emotions. Research has proved that expression of anger and hostility can play an important role in modifying disease progression. Bottled up emotions can play havoc on many vital systems in the body. Exercise provides a socially acceptable means of physically releasing these bottled up feelings. As you are smashing balls on the squash court, you are not just burning calories or letting out sweat, you are also unknowingly releasing a lot of anger in a healthy way.

Exercise: A Meditation in Motion

Certain exercises like aerobic dance, jogging, swimming, hiking, bicycling, which require a fairly consistent repetitive motion, can alter one's state of consciousness. This state is very similar to what has been attained during dynamic meditation leading some beneficiaries to describe it as a moving meditation. The physiological effects of exercising are very similar to what happens when one practices meditation. Both induce deep breathing, act as a tranquilizer and produce feelings of calmness, deep within.

Exercise: A Boost to Social Life

Exercising, especially outside the confines of your home, can give a boost to your social life. It gives you an opportunity to meet new people, draw inspiration from each other and even expand your social network. This can effectively abate stress in your life. Further, exercise adds spice to life and drives away boredom. Too little stress

CHAPTER 22 : EXERCISE - A POTENT STRESS BUSTER

in one's life can be just as upsetting as too much stress. It is natural for humans to seek out some stimulation and excitement. For some the opportunity for physical challenges is the most interesting part of life. This urge can be expressed through activities, such as running as fast as one can, swimming as far as one can, or hitting a golf ball as straight and long as possible. We like to set challenging mini goals for ourselves to create excitement. On the far end of the spectrum there are people who voluntarily involve themselves in high-risk physical activities such as extreme skiing, hang gliding, scuba diving, and skydiving. By constantly testing our limits, we learn how to take on higher and higher loads of stress. Mind you, this is the enjoyable form of stress, or Eustress. This phenomenon is quite similar to using counter irritant to kill an original irritant. A balm that stings makes us forget the original pain. Here too the stress encountered in these challenging, adrenalin activities replaces the real life stress and teaches the person how to deal with it effectively.

Exercise: Fights Insomnia
Stress is the enemy of sleep. Stress overload for some is the cause of insomnia. Inability to sleep or get adequate rest creates further stress and the vicious cycle continues. A sleep deprived, fatigued individual is less able to perform at a high level. Exercise has been shown to be very effective in helping some individuals fall asleep easily and sleep more soundly. Exercise ensures better quality and depth of sleep, which can energize you to face the stresses of life better.

Exercise: Fitter to Fight Disease
One who is physically fit and has his physical system functioning at an optimal level can evade common place ailments. Exercising helps build this immunity. Those who exercise demonstrate more stamina and greater resiliency to fight the discomfort. They are also likely to recover more quickly.

Exercise: Ushers Quality Time with Self
Exercise allows you the luxury of spending quality time with

yourself. It can be an escape from the daily toils and pressures of a stressful society. All form of exercises, from an invigorating walk to a bicycle ride, swimming laps in a pool to an early morning run, all these activities allow you to recharge your creative batteries. It gives you time to be with your own thoughts, introspect, even indulge in some motivating self-talk.

HOW TO EXERCISE: THE SWAN FORMULA
The components of exercise can be remembered if you keep in mind the SWAN formula.

SWAN is a mnemonic which makes remembering facts easy. I introduced this formula in my book titled *REAL fitness*. In fact, REAL is itself a mnemonic which includes Relaxation, Exercise, Attitude and Laughter.

Welcome to the SWAN formula:
- S for stretching
- W for weight training
- A for aerobics, and
- N for nutrition.

I have included nutrition in the SWAN formula, as nutrition and exercise go hand in hand; one is incomplete without the other if REAL fitness is desired. After all, nutrition is very much a form of exercise — an exercise of control.

For more detailed information on exercise and nutrition you could refer to *REAL Fitness* published by Marine sport.

> Exercise not only gives us a beautiful body, it gives us a peaceful mind too. The stress hormones are effectively neutralized by exercise just as our health improves and diseases are kept at bay.

Stretching

CHAPTER 23

Calm Sutra views stretching or flexibility training as a very pleasurable stress-buster. As you stretch your body you can feel a sense of well-being engulf you. As you focus your awareness on the muscle being stretched you are consumed by the present, with no opportunity for worry.

Stretching is one of the most essential exercises to increase flexibility and reduce injuries. Stretching exercises include movements like forward-bending, toe-touching, wall push-ups and other movements which elongate muscles and improve joint motion. Stretching is a must before and after aerobic exercise or weight training. Stretching can also be done by itself to release all the tensions in the muscles. It is a great way to begin a day. Stretching exercises are a must for persons working on the computer to rid the stiffness caused by sitting for hours in front of the machine. Most of the stretches are similar to the asanas taught in Yoga.

Sportspersons cannot do without stretching. It is an essential pre-requisite to make the muscles, joints and all the connective tissue flexible before starting the sport. Lack of flexibility can have disastrous consequences for a sportsperson. Sprains, muscle pulls, ligament tears and tendon ruptures are associated with poor flexibility. Competitive sport can have quite an unbalancing effect on

> If you do not stretch your muscles, you are stretching your luck. Stretch or the stretcher, the choice is yours.
> *Baba Calm Dev*

the body. Take racket sports for example. The same arm is used to hit thousands of shots over and over again. One side of the body is placed under different types and levels of stress compared to the other. A flexibility training programme can help to correct these disparities preventing chronic, over-use injury.

Of course, a more flexible athlete is a more mobile athlete. It allows enhanced movement around the court or field with greater ease and dexterity. Recreational sportspersons should follow the same stretching routine that the professionals follow, if they would like to avoid injury.

I was lucky to be a member of a Vyayamshala, an ethnic Indian gymnasium as a kid. Great emphasis was placed on flexibility training or stretching exercises at the Vyayamshala. The Suryanamaskar or the Sun salutation is an example of a comprehensive stretching programme for the entire body. I would recommend you to learn the Suryanamaskar to enhance your flexibility and overall fitness.

WHY ARE SOME PEOPLE MORE FLEXIBLE THAN OTHERS?

A lot of stress is created when one compares one's flexibility levels with others, especially in the gym. The feeling of 'I am trying so hard and yet I can't touch my nose to the knees like her' is quite common. A number of anatomical and physiological factors influence a person's flexibility.

Inherent Joint Structure

There are different types of joints in the human body. Some intrinsically have a greater range of motion like the shoulder, which is a ball and socket joint. The shoulder is more flexible than the knee, which is a modified hinge.

Age and Gender

It is well-known that flexibility decreases with age. This is due, in part to the fibrous connective tissue that replace muscle fibres

CHAPTER 23 : STRETCHING

through a process called fibrosis. Older individuals should take encouragement that, just as with strength and endurance, flexibility can be increased at any age with training.

Generally, females tend to be more flexible than males, physically at least!

Ligaments and Tendons

Ligaments and tendons do not seem to display any elastic properties. However, with exposure to stretching they may slightly extend to a new length. One must also remember that increased mobility in the ligaments reduces the stability of the joint, which is not welcome.

Muscle Bulk and Weight Training

Increase in muscle bulk or hypertrophy of skeletal muscle can adversely affect the flexibility or the range of motion. It may be difficult for bulky athletes to complete certain stretches, such as an overhead triceps stretch or assume the stork position. However, a stretch and strengthen programme can ensure range along with strength, for better function.

Temperature and Sleep

The athlete's internal environment affects the Range Of Motion or ROM. For example, mobility is decreased immediately upon waking after a night's sleep. Ten minutes in a warm (40°C) bath increases body temperature and ROM.

Previous Injury

Many times injuries to muscles heal with a process called fibrosis, which can reduce the elasticity of the muscle. This is true with most injuries to connective tissues. Fibrous tissue is less elastic and can lead to muscle shortening and reduced ROM. A massage technique called myo-fascial release may be able to alleviate pain and restriction caused by trigger points.

BENEFITS OF STRETCHING

Stretching exercises should form an integral part of any conditioning programme. Performed consistently, the stretching exercises below can help to do the following:

- Increase the range of motion about a joint reducing the risk of muscle and tendon tears during sporting activity.
- Relieve muscle tightness and stiffness.
- Improve postural imbalances and help to reduce chronic back pain.
- Increase localized blood flow to the muscles being stretched.
- Possibly relieve muscle soreness after intense physical activity and help to reduce the severity of DOMS (Delayed Onset Muscle Soreness).
- Help relieve pain and stiffness caused by prolonged activities like sitting at a computer or deejaying.
- And above all, stretching exercise is a stress-buster by itself. When you stretch with awareness, you are enjoying the moment thoroughly.

TYPES OF STRETCHING EXERCISES

There are two types of stretching: Static and Dynamic. In the former, a muscle is slowly stretched and held in the lengthened position for a period of time. Each specific stretch position is held for 20 to 30 seconds. During this period, one focuses on the muscle being stretched. The feeling of the slight tension in the stretching muscle should slowly subside. Then one stretches a bit further until the mild tension is felt again. There should never be any pain felt during stretching.

In Dynamic Stretching, the muscles are stretched, while in motion. Dynamic stretch is a controlled form of rehearsal of the specific movements, which are to follow in a workout or in a sporting activity. Dynamic stretches are performed after static stretches. For example, a person before playing tennis will do warm up, static stretches and then dynamic stretches before starting the game. The dynamic stretches will include slow forehand and backhand movements and overhead movements, similar to the physical exercises that are to follow.

STRETCHING TIPS

- Always warm up before stretching. Warming up gives your body a chance to deliver plenty of nutrient rich blood to areas about to be exercised, which warms the muscles and lubricates the joints.
- Do not bounce or bob when you stretch — not only is this not effective, but you could injure yourself.
- Take each stretch slowly to the point where tension can be felt, but not pain.
- Never stretch torn or injured muscles unless you have consulted your doctor.
- Hold each stretch for 20 to 30 seconds.
- Always complete each stretch for both sides of your body, when applicable.
- Always cool down and relax after a stretching session. By cooling down, you can help prevent injuries and muscle soreness from your workout.

> Stretching is a great way of improving flexibility and minimizing injury to our muscles and joints. Stretching, if performed mindfully and with awareness, can be a great way of enjoying the moment and feeling good.

CHAPTER 24

Weight Training

An Ode to the Muscle:
Oh my muscle, my buddy, my chum,
You make me run; make me have all the fun,
You give a curve to my bum and metabolize all the rum,
Tara rum pum tara rum pum…
(Hip Hop beat)

> Training gives us an outlet for suppressed energies created by stress and thus tones the spirit just as exercise conditions the body
> *Arnold Schwarzenegger*

Weight training is a very effective stress-buster. The action of weightlifting itself is quite gratifying. It instantly elevates the mood, while filling the self with a sense of achievement. The visible cosmetic results and health benefits are a bonus.

When we workout using weights or resistance we are utilizing one of the most important, yet underrated systems in the body, i.e., the muscular system. The muscles we exercise are called voluntary muscles. They are completely obedient and listen to every command we make to them. We need them when we want to walk, to swim, to pick up a glass of water, to breathe etc. If we want to exercise we use them, if we want to burn fat we use them, to play sports we use them, to protect our joints we need them and they obey us making very few demands. Even at rest these muscles are burning calories and take active part in the metabolism. In return we can express our gratitude by exercising them, stretching them, giving them nutritious

CHAPTER 24 : WEIGHT TRAINING

food and occasionally massaging them, so that they continue with their job tirelessly.

Weight training is a generic term for all exercises that develop the strength and size of voluntary muscles. There are many different methods of weight training; the most common being the use of weights against gravity. One can choose between weights like dumb-bells and barbells or pulley systems or you can use your own body weight as resistance. Weight training is included in the group of exercises called strength training which includes resistance training where elastic or hydraulic forces are used to oppose muscle contraction.

Properly performed, weight training can provide significant functional benefits and improvement in overall health and well-being including increased bone, muscle, tendon and ligament strength and toughness, improved joint function, reduced potential for injury, improved cardiac function and elevated levels of good cholesterol. The posture also improves which improves breathing capacity. The looks improve because of fat loss and better muscle definition, and all of this put together improves the confidence and self-esteem.

Weight training when performed with awareness results in reduction of stress. When the mind focuses on the muscle being worked out, it is forced to be in the moment. A great deal of intrinsic happiness can be derived by working out with full awareness. Apart from the mind being in sync with the muscle, the mirror(usually kept all around training zones) can also be used to great benefit while training with weights. The mirror is not an instrument for narcissism but a device to help you remain aware of your body posture or form while you enjoy the workout.

HISTORY OF WEIGHT TRAINING

Hippocrates explained the principle behind strength training when he wrote "that which is used develops, and that which is not used wastes away". This simply translates to 'use it or lose it'. Muscles which are not used shrink at an alarming rate, known as disuse atrophy.

Progressive Resistance Training traces its roots to ancient Greece.

Legend has it that wrestler Milo of Croton, trained by carrying a newborn calf on his back every day until it was fully grown. His muscles adapted to the growth of the calf, by growing themselves, till he was able to achieve the feat of carrying a full grown bull.

Strength training became increasingly popular in the 1980s, following the release of the bodybuilding movie 'Pumping Iron' and the subsequent popularity of Arnold Schwarzenegger. Strength training is no longer an exclusive domain of males as more and more women are resorting to it, the world over.

ADVANTAGES OF WEIGHT TRAINING

With weight training exercises, one builds up muscles which increases one's resting metabolic rate and provide the individual with the necessary fuel involved in calorie burning. They also build muscle endurance. Circuit weight training, for example, are a set of exercises aimed at building muscle endurance. All types of aerobic exercises which burn calories and fat during a workout also do the same.

Weight training is also helpful in burning fat. Heavyweight training is responsible in burning fat. When a muscle is rebuilt after a workout, there are certain hormones, which are secreted. These hormones contribute to growth of the muscles by redirecting fat from the depot areas to the muscle areas.

Stronger muscles prevent degeneration of joints and help in conditions like osteoporosis. So weight training contributes to prevention of joint related disorders. A person with stronger muscles is less likely to get disorders like tennis elbow and spondylosis. A person with better muscles can withstand an injury better with minimal damage to the tissues.

Strength training improves posture and personality in general. It improves performance in the field of sports and also reduces the chances of injury.

USE OF EQUIPMENT IN WEIGHT TRAINING

A wide variety of equipment has been used in weight training. The most popular are dumb-bells. I personally enjoy and recommend

CHAPTER 24 : WEIGHT TRAINING

weight-training exercises with a pair of light dumb-bells. With proper technique most of the muscles in the body can be strengthened with the use of dumb-bells. The main advantage of dumb-bells is that they are cheap and can be used in a small area.

Pulley machines have revolutionarized weight training. Though they are bulky, the pulley system is the least injurious of the weight training methods. There are very few compressive stresses on the joints and the machines work on distraction principles.

Strength training using one's own body weight is termed as Free Hand Muscle Toning. The popular exercises using this principle are squats, sit-ups, pull-ups, push-ups, etc. The advantage is their convenience and simplicity. The problem with this type of training is that overweight people can cause injuries to their muscles and joints due to overloading by their excessive body weight. Persons using weights like dumb-bells and pulleys avoid these injuries by choosing weights that are much lighter.

TIPS FOR STRESS-FREE WEIGHT TRAINING

- Concentrate on the muscles while exercising. Focus on the muscle group which is being exercised.
- Maintain a good rhythm during exercise. Lift slowly for 2 seconds (positive stroke) and 4 seconds for getting back to the starting position (negative stroke). Repeat this procedure in a rhythm.
- Knees and elbows should be soft during most exercises, meaning that the knee and elbow joints are never to be fully extended during the exercises so as to protect them from injury.
- Exhale during the positive stroke or exertion and inhale during the negative stroke.
- Start light and then work your way up. Always begin with smaller weights.
- Start with larger muscles and then work the smaller ones. Bench press before curls.
- Rest between sets for 30 to 60 seconds and then begin the

new set.
- Rest for 48 hours between workouts to help muscles recover.
- Take professional help to chalk out your programme and to teach you the correct technique.
- Warm up and stretch before the work out and cool down after weight training.

> Weight training, if properly performed, can provide significant functional benefits apart from making us look and feel better. There is overall improvement in health and well-being with weight training, which includes increased bone, muscle and improved joint function, reduced potential for injury and better posture.

Aerobic Exercise

CHAPTER 25

Aerobic exercise is one of the integral parts of Calm Sutra, which gives great stress release along with comprehensive health benefits.

Aerobic exercise or cardio training comprises of a prolonged set of repetitive movements that is usually set to a rhythm. It utilizes oxygen from the atmosphere, burns calories and gives workout to your cardiovascular system. Aerobic exercises makes you more fitter as well as a more positive and happier person.

Every minute of your life whether awake or asleep, your body is burning fuel to produce energy. Whether you undertake an activity like walking briskly or climbing a few flights of stairs you need more energy. The muscles in our body need more oxygen, along with the carbohydrate for proper functioning, especially in emergencies brought on by stress or by indulging in rigorous workouts.

The purpose of aerobic activity is to improve the delivery of oxygen to the muscles. This, in turn, would make muscles more strong and capable of producing energy. The benefits of aerobic exercise are enormous and include weight loss, increase in life expectancy and an enhanced feeling of well-being.

> Aerobic exercise is 100 per cent inspiration and perspiration.
> *Baba Calm Dev*

WHAT ARE THE TYPES OF AEROBIC EXERCISES?

Aerobic exercise was introduced by Kenneth Cooper and popularized by Jane Fonda. For a long time aerobics was associated with young girls dancing to the beat of music. This is but half-truth. Aerobic exercise includes any activity like brisk walking, jogging, swimming, or games like squash, tennis, which utilize the oxygen from the atmosphere to burn calories. Activities like circuit weight training, where one lifts light weights for many repetitions are also included in aerobic exercise.

THE F.I.T. OF AEROBICS

If one wants the best benefits from aerobic exercise it is essential to remember the F.I.T. principle.

F.I.T. stands for Frequency, Intensity, and Time.

Frequency

For an aerobic exercise to be effective and safe it is essential that the frequency of aerobic exercise be optimum. It is recommended that 3 to 4 days of aerobic exercise per week results in excellent cardio-vascular benefits and fat loss. Exercising every day may be harmful and the benefits may not be more in comparison to the 3 - 4 day workout schedule. On the other hand, exercising once or twice a week may not be adequate for reaping good benefits from an aerobic programme. Hence an optimality ought to be maintained.

Intensity

Intensity is the most important factor to be kept in mind when one is performing aerobic exercises. The intensity must be adequate to get the desired results and should not exceed physiological limits and invite stress, strain and injury. To monitor the intensity of aerobic exercise, the pulse rate is considered a good guide.

Training Zone or Target Heart Rate

To find out the target heart rate zone, one applies a very simple formula. While exercising, your pulse rate must be in a range of 60-80 per cent of your maximal heart rate. The maximal heart rate is the difference between the number 220 and your age. Your pulse

CHAPTER 25 : AEROBIC EXERCISE

rate during the workouts should correspond to 60-80 per cent of this figure. It has been seen that persons who workout with their heart rate near the 60 per cent mark have great results in fat burning. However, the persons working out at the upper end of the training zone have better results with cardiovascular enhancement.

There are other ways to assess if the level of exercise is optimal or not. Look for signs of breathlessness, fatigue and inability to talk after a workout. The intensity of your workout is very high if you find it difficult to complete a sentence without pausing for breath. It is also too mild in intensity if you can sing during exercise.

Time

The next question a person doing aerobic exercise faces is how long should an aerobic exercise programme last. For lasting benefits of aerobic exercise on the cardiovascular system and reduction of fat, 30-45 minutes of aerobic exercise programme is essential. Also, it is useful to know the ideal time for exercising. Generally, mornings are considered better, as the post exercise benefits of aerobic exercise are derived best from morning sessions. The body is propelled into a higher metabolic state early in the morning and this is continued through a large part of the day. Even after cessation of exercise, the body continues to burn calories, which are extremely helpful for those on a weight reduction programme. The concentration and creativity levels are also very high after a workout in the morning. An early morning session further recharges your battery, gives a feel-good attitude and makes one confident and spirited.

AEROBIC LIFESTYLE

A lot of people have incorporated certain lifestyle changes so as to remain fit and healthy. It is not always possible to have a regimented fitness programme. However, this is not an excuse they see to escape workouts. Throughout the day they indulge in their diurnal activities and look for ways within their bust schedules to shave off calories. This is a very proactive way of thinking and for

CALM SUTRA : THE ART OF RELAXATION

such people unavoidable exertion is bonus exercise.
Some of the lifestyle changes you can opt for are:

- Take the stairs instead of elevators.
- Walk to and from the market.
- Involve yourself in household activities like tiding up, dusting, sweeping, swabbing, cleaning, mowing the lawn, etc.
- Wear shoes with laces, tying them will help you maintain flexibility.
- Do not use the remote control for television, walk to the television to switch channels.
- If you have a choice then sit instead of lying down, stand instead of sitting, walk instead of standing, climb instead of walking.

SAFE AEROBIC EXERCISES

It is very essential that aerobic exercises be made enjoyable and free from stress, strain and injury. The various aerobic exercises can be broadly divided into low impact and high impact exercises depending on the amount of calories that is being burnt.

The low impact exercises include walking, swimming, cycling and games like golf which do not involve too much of running around. So, low impact aerobic exercises are more spaced out and are less likely to cause overstrain.

Jogging, running, playing tennis and squash form the high impact exercise group. Aerobic dance itself can be high impact or low impact depending upon the steps involved. High impact aerobic dance involves a lot of jumping and bouncing. Low impact aerobic dances have one foot rooted to the ground and the movements are milder.

High impact aerobic exercise, though found to be more thrilling and fulfilling, does pose a lot of stress to the feet, ankles, knees and spine. All beginners must start with low impact exercises and once the body is conditioned to the schedule and form of exercises then only should the switch to high impact exercises take place.

However, brisk walking is really the best form of aerobic exercise,

CHAPTER 25 : AEROBIC EXERCISE

as it gives all the benefits of jogging and poses very few chances of injury. Persons with knee or back problems, who desire weight loss and cardiovascular fitness are usually advised stationary cycling or swimming, as these are some of the safest forms of aerobic exercise.

PRECAUTIONS TO BE FOLLOWED

To add more safety to aerobic exercise, one should never forget to warm up and stretch the body before exercise. Equally important is to cool down at the end of it all. One must pay attention to the footwear. Wear shoes that give you a good grip and bounce and also something that is light weight. The market is flooded with footwear designed for exercising and it is advisable to use them.

It is also important to pay attention to the surface on which exercise is done. A rough, uneven surface could mean bad news for the joints and muscles.

With these precautions in place, aerobic exercises can be great fun and have an enormous bounty of health benefits for the individual.

LAUNCH AGAINST THE PAUNCH WITH AEROBIC EXERCISE

Waist management is vital — Baba Calm Dev

The media has assailed our senses with men and women having perfect figures and complete with washboard abdomens. Fat around the waist is a complete no, when it comes to current definitions of beauty and perhaps this is why more and more people are in the pursuit for that flat abdomen and stomach. Gym instructors are under pressure to devise ways of getting the perfect figure for their clients, essentially flattened stomachs for their clients. Health equipment manufacturers are into bringing out fancy devices which promise to deflate the pot belly. People are taking to vibrators and tummy trimmers and are willing to spend a lot of money in the pursuit of a paunchless figure.

Baba Calm Dev has a story to tell.

It is about Aesop's hare and the tortoise. Years later, the hare and tortoise both developed paunches and heartily disliked it. They decided to have a race. This time it would be around who could lose his paunch first.

The hare was sold out on the commercials that he saw on the television and bought himself a fancy tummy trimmer. The hare performed crunches and abdominal sit-ups with this equipment and worked really hard.

The tortoise, a firm believer of Calm Sutra walked, swam, cycled and he even played golf. He paid attention to his diet, ate sensibly and drank a lot of water.

All the while the hare laughed at him.

On judgment day the tortoise arrived minus his paunch. He had burnt his flab quicker. The hare still had a long way to go. Once again the tortoise beat the hare. Once again, it was a bad hare day, says Baba Calm Dev.

The moral of the story is that mere abdominal exercises will not be able to reduce the fat around the stomach. In fact, it is to be complemented with a proper diet, hydrotherapy and a positive frame of mind.

Why abdominal exercises alone will NOT reduce my paunch?

There is a fair amount of literature on ways to tackle the bulge, especially around the midriff. A lot of fat trimming machines have been launched in the market; various crunches, sit-ups and abdominal exercises have been advocated. However, none of them on their own have led to the desired results.

What actually works is a combination of aerobic exercise and diet.

Let us begin with the fundamental question as to what is the paunch? A paunch is the much used term for the collection of fat around the waist giving rise to the pear-shaped body. This fat can be subcutaneous (under the skin) or intra-abdominal (inside the abdominal wall around the organs).

Midriff Fat (MRF) causes a paunch. MRF will not be melted by just performing any amount of abdominal exercises. This fat needs to be cut off by increasing the metabolic rate. Aerobic exercises can help a lot in raising this level. The fat from the waist is mobilized

CHAPTER 25 : AEROBIC EXERCISE

and converted into fuel during aerobic exercise. Alongside a negative calorie balance is created with proper diet and aerobic exercise. A kilo of waist fat needs a calorie deficit of about 7000 calories. So, a proper diet is a must when one is on a weight and fat reduction programme especially through aerobic exercises.

For burning just one kg of waist fat, the abdominal muscles will have to create an output of 7000 calories and for that you would have to perform about 10 thousand sit-ups!

I have seen a lot of overuse injuries in people resorting to excessive abdominal exercises and still not achieving any appreciable fat loss. Therefore the moot question that arises here is: Are abdominal exercises and crunches absolutely useless?

ABDOMINAL EXERCISES : THE REAL FACTS

The answer to the above question is that abdominal exercises are not completely useless or unnecessary. However, stand alone, they may not be able to do much. They may not burn fat but they sure would be able to give you a great muscular and toned body. Further, it has the potential to improve your posture and prevent back problems. Abdominal exercises will help you develop fabulous abdominal muscles called a six pack, which resemble biscuits or a chocolate slab! These exercises are useful after pregnancy and certain abdominal operations to regain the muscle tone at your waist. Abdominal workouts do not burn fat and hence they are not really apt for a fat loss programme.

Core Strength and Good Posture

If you have been following the trends in exercise and fitness, you probably must have heard the phrase 'core strength'. Core strength refers to the muscles of your abdomen and back and their ability to support your spine and keep your body stable and balanced. Good core strength keeps the back strong and can prevent backache and many degenerative conditions like spondylosis. If you are a golfer or a tennis player it is vital to have good core strength. Your power will increase and the chances of injury are minimized.

Core Muscles

The major muscles of your core include the four abdominal muscles and the main back extensor muscle.

The main abdominal muscles include TVA or the transverses abdomini, internal and external obliques and the rectus abdomini or the six pack muscle. The problem with those who do crunches is that they only exercise the rectus abdomini and leave out the rest. For good core strength exercises like the plank, arm sweeps and crossover crunches are needed. To strengthen the back extensor or the erector spinae muscles, back extensions on a roman chair and Yoga asanas like the Bhujangasana or the Cobra Pose should be done.

So remember there is more to your abdomen than a sexy six pack.

Wishing you happy waist management.

Aerobic exercise improves cardiac function and facilitates fat loss enjoyably. Aerobic exercises should be performed with right intensity, frequency and duration for optimum benefits including stress release.

CHAPTER 26

Walking Away from Stress

"No I don't exercise, I just walk," is a common answer I get when I ask my patients about their fitness routine. People often think nothing about the immense benefits they derive from walking. They take walking for granted and forget that it is one of the best forms of exercise for the body and mind.

Walking is possibly the least complicated, safest, cheapest and enjoyable road to fitness, good health and happiness.

Walking is recognized as a proven modality to fight stress and its ill effects. You can literally walk away from your worries and leave them far behind.

Walking, apart from being the most basic form of transport for the human being, can produce a variety of sensations depending on the location and pace of your walk. The intensity of walking can range from a leisurely after-dinner stroll, to frantic race walking. It can be a power walk where you can get the benefit of an aerobic exercise or it can be of spiritual value like in a labyrinth walk. It can be a community walk to spread peace or AIDS awareness or it can be a very personal introspective walk. You can have a creative walk where you can compose music or write poetry or walk 18 holes while playing golf. Yes, you can choose your style and the pace of your walk, and whichever way you do it,

> All truly great thoughts are conceived while walking.
> *Friedrich Nietzsche*

walking does enrich your life in more ways than one.

BENEFITS OF WALKING

There are numerous health benefits of walking as it is a weight bearing, low impact aerobic exercise with many pleasures and few perils. Persons with severe osteoarthritis of the knees or spine and those with advanced heart problems need to be cautious while resorting to walking as an exercise.

Cardio Vascular Benefits

The heart benefits a lot from walking. Numerous studies have shown that walking can control and reverse coronary artery disease. Walking directly affects the heart by increasing its output and function.

Walking reduces the coronary risk factors by reducing blood lipids like cholesterol and controlling hypertension. Patients with proven heart disease may well be able to avoid major heart surgeries by taking up walking as a part of their daily routine.

Fat Burn

Even a moderate intensity walk can help in fat burn. If you raise your heart beat rate to just above 60 percent of maximum heart rate and maintain it for about 45 minutes you will notice appreciable fat loss. Fats are mobilized from their depot areas and converted to ready energy required for the walk. A good paced walk can burn more than 300 Cals in an hour.

Control of Diseases

Diseases like diabetes mellitus can be controlled by brisk walking. Several patients with diabetes have successfully cut down on their drug dosage, even become drug free after resorting to regular brisk walking. However, this ought to be supported with a proper diet programme. A study reported in the *Annals of Internal Medicine* suggested that, increased physical activity, including regular walking, substantially reduced risk for cardiovascular events in diabetic women.

Maintains Posture

Once you adopt the correct style of walking, the posture in general improves. The muscles involved in maintaining a healthy erect posture are given a good drill during walking. The alignment of the head, spine and limbs is maintained and even the core muscles are given a work out. Walking if done with complete awareness maintains proper posture and affects one's grace and overall appearance.

Provides a Total Body Workout

Walking is not an exercise for the lower extremities alone. Walking, while exercising the prime movers like the calves, the thigh and the hip muscles, involves almost every muscle in the body. The arms are swinging, the back and neck muscles are involved too as are the shoulders and the head. Hence it is good for every conceivable part of the body.

Deep breathing, which is needed to enrich your blood with oxygen while walking, gives the abdominal muscles and the diaphragm to chance to work at their best capacity.

Osteoporosis Reduced

Research has shown that bone density can be improved with walking. Of course calcium, vitamin D and hormonal balance are also necessary to fight osteoporosis but the value of walking cannot be overlooked. Walking is a weight bearing exercise, where the large bones of the lower extremities take the load of the body. This along with the muscle action of the calf and thigh muscles stimulates formation of bone mass. If the walk is outdoors the gentle sunshine can add to the stronger bone formation.

Less Injury

Though walking is a weight bearing exercise, it does not put much impact on the joints, unlike jogging and running. The main reason for walking being a low impact exercise is due to the fact that one foot is always on the ground. This ensures that there is no undue

CALM SUTRA : THE ART OF RELAXATION

strain on the joints and the cartilages. As an orthopaedic surgeon I see very few injuries arising from walking, be it brisk walking, power walking or even the high-speed race walking.

Really Affordable

Walking can be truly termed as a common man's exercise. You do not need to be a member of any exclusive club, there are no coaching fees, you don't have to get expensive equipment or pay any membership fees. All you need is a good pair of walking shoes and a desire in your heart. As long as you wear good footwear the surface does not matter much. You could walk on the road, in a park or on the beach. If you are lucky and have a community walking track, do make the most of it.

Anti Stress

Walking can help relieve stress. A study published in the Annals of Behavioural Medicine on Nov. 9, 1999 showed that university students, who walked or did other forms of moderate exercise regularly, had lower stress levels as opposed to those who did not exercise at all or those who indulged in too rigourous fitness schedules.

Walking gives you time to think, as well as time to get away from the stressors. Getting out of the stressful environment, breathing the air and feeling your body move is natural stress-relief. With walking you put a physical and mental distance between yourself and the stress-causing environment which can in turn promote objectivity towards the stressful event. People often return from their walks recharged and refreshed and with fresher insights. Walking gives you a chance to feel your body in motion the same way that one can feel one's movements during dynamic meditation.

You can enjoy the environment around you and perform green meditation. You can proactively plan the day ahead and chart out a schedule. You can talk and laugh with your walking partner to relieve the stress. When walking, in a group or otherwise, apart from the very tangible health benefits, there are enormous other benefits

CHAPTER 26 : WALKING AWAY FROM STRESS

too which can help a person grow in a more positive direction. Therefore it is a good stress busting, physically invigorating measure that needs little investment apart from time from the individual and hence should be on top of the agenda for most of us.

HOW TO WALK

Though walking is a low impact exercise, one needs to walk correctly to enjoy greater benefits and fewer problems. The posture, which involves head position, spine and limb alignment, is very important. The other important factors involved are stride length, arm movement and dynamics of the feet when they make contact with the ground. With simple tips the walk can help you burn more calories and give you a make-over that is both on the outside as well as inside.

The Pre Walk Routine

The pre-walk routine requires warm up and a few stretching exercises. The warm up can be achieved by a few minutes of spot walking or walking slowly to the starting point of your regular track.

Stretching is extremely important to avoid injury and make your walk more enjoyable. The calf muscles, the front leg muscles, the quadriceps, the hamstring and the hip muscles should be stretched. Since the entire body is also involved in the walk do not forget to stretch the arms, the forearms, the neck and the back muscles.

The Tall-walker Posture

If you walk with awareness you will derive greater benefits from your walk. The awareness will prompt action, which will help you improve your posture and style of walking. Good walking posture will help you diminish the few injuries associated with walking.

Think tall and walk tall. That is the mantra to be followed while walking. Imagine a painless hook going through your scalp which applies traction and elongates your body. Stand erect and pull yourself till that height. Remember it is not a military march nor is

CALM SUTRA : THE ART OF RELAXATION

it a slouched amble. It is a relaxed yet erect and graceful walk.

1. Be as erect as possible.
2. Think of being tall and straight,
3. Do not arch your back.
4. Do not lean forward or lean back. Leaning puts strain on the back muscles.
5. Eyes forward, try to spot a pothole 20 feet ahead!
6. Keep the chin parallel to the ground. This relaxes the neck muscles.
7. Think shoulders to be wide and slightly back, but not military.
8. Gently tuck in your stomach.

Involve your Upper Body

The upper body actively takes part in the walk. The proper use of the upper body can help you burn more calories and exercise more muscles of the body when you walk. There should be no tension in the arms and the fists should not be clenched tightly to avoid elevating your blood pressure.

1. Bend your elbows a little less than 90 degrees.
2. Hands should be closed in a loose manner, do not clench into a tight fist.
3. As you stride, the arm opposite your forward foot should come straight forward.
4. The arms should swing close to your body in a straight line front and back.
5. The arc of the arm swing should be up to your mid-chest level.

The "Heel to Toe" Stride

Walking involves an easy rolling motion where the entire foot takes part in the forward propulsion of the body. I have been a habitual toe walker all my life and I have to make conscious effort to use my feet correctly. Remember...

1. The heel strikes the ground first.
2. The body weight is gently transferred forward from heel to toe.
3. Final push off is effected by the great toe.

CHAPTER 26 : WALKING AWAY FROM STRESS

4. The same sequence of heel strike, forward roll and toe push off is repeated.
5. Good walking shoes are flexible and they ensure the roll through action.
6. In an attempt to increase speed do not over-stride, you could pull some muscle.
7. To increase your speed, take smaller and quicker steps.

GOOD SHOES FOR STRESS-FREE WALKING

Good shoes are necessary for deriving the best benefits from walking. For people who ask me for shoe recommendations, my advice is, "please use walking shoes for walking and not tennis shoes or slippers for walking".

Shoe companies have spent a great deal of money in designing various shoes for various activities. A lot of research has gone into making these shoes. The 'sports shoes' is a broad generic term. In fact they are meant to be more specific in their actions. Sports shoes today, are activity specific and designed for better performance. They look at the safety aspects for that particular sporting activity. A running shoe is different from a walking shoe, which is completely different from a tennis shoe as they cater to different forms of sports or activities. A sports shoe is your ally in getting the best from your sport and you ought to be making a health statement in them, not a fashion statement.

As for selecting walking shoes, I don't like to make specific shoe recommendations because everyone's foot is different and people have different walking styles. But there are a few basic points to remember while selecting walking shoes:

Look for a low, supportive heel that does not flair out. A thick heel will cause your foot to slap down rather than roll. This slows down forward momentum and increases the occurrence of sore shins.

For correct and smooth weight transfer from heel to toe, a flexible sole is better. It needs to bend more in the toe than a runner. You should be able to twist and bend the toe area.

Next, look for a shoe that is light weight and breathable. The last thing you want is the clunky heavy leather walking shoe.

The fit is most important factor in the walking shoe. Be sure your foot has enough room in the toe box. There should be about a centimeter gap between your toes and the end of the shoe. The shoe should be wide enough in the toe so that your toes can move freely. Your heel should be snug and should not slip. The shoe should not pinch or strangulate your foot anywhere.

Shoe shopping should be done at the end of the day or after your walk when your feet may be slightly swollen. Also be sure to wear the same socks you will be wearing during your walks. This can make a huge difference in how the shoe fits. Try on both shoes. Your feet may not be the same size.

Discard the shoe when they have lost their bounce rather than when they are worn out. The walking shoes usually lose their cushioning after 600 kilometers. This is the time to change them.

WALKING WITH GOD

A few years back, we took a trip to the shrine of Vaishnodevi, in the state of Jammu and Kashmir. Vaishnodevi is a very popular place of pilgrimage for the Hindus. On the trek to Vaishnodevi I encountered God. I met God many times during the 14 km uphill walk. God came in the shape of the cool breeze which hit my face, the refreshing water I drank, the beautiful mountains and valleys I saw, the rhythmic melodious chants I heard, and the lovely people I was walking with. We were supposed to meet God at peak, but for me God was walking by my side, all the time.

> Walking is possibly the least complicated, safest, cheapest and an enjoyable way to fitness, good health and happiness. Walking performed with awareness can be meditative.

Running to De-Stress

CHAPTER 27

Former US president Jimmy Carter says, "Anyone who has run knows that its most important value is in removing tension and allowing a release from whatever other cares the day may bring".

A person who does not run will never understand the joys of running. The vast majority perceive it as painful, tedious and exhausting. So why do so many people run? People run for various reasons. Most often, people run to stay in shape and to reach an ideal body weight. Others run to keep their sugars or cholesterols in check. Some run as a matter of routine and others run for the love of it.

The ones who have tasted the runner's high soon get addicted and do not like to miss their daily fix. I remember the case of India's leading marathon runner, Shivkumar Yadav. He had sustained a knee injury for which we had performed a ligament reconstruction surgery. The surgery required rest for 6 weeks and running was absolutely forbidden. Shivkumar was like a fish out of water without his running regime and would beg and plead with us to let him off. We had a hard time pacifying him.

Dr Sanjay Pai, an eminent orthopaedic surgeon from Bangalore runs every morning and is addicted to it. For Sanjay running is not just health management, it is a source of ultimate bliss for him.

> Running a marathon is like running a company: You are the CEO, your mind is the capital; your heart, lungs, limbs are your employees; your preparation, your exercise and your diet are the investment; and "high" is the dividend.
>
> *Baba Calm Dev*

Anil Ambani, India's leading industrialist runs an empire. He runs first thing in the morning and then attends to his vast business empire, later in the day. I have seen the euphoria on his face as he finishes his morning run. What started as a weight management programme for Mr. Ambani is now a passion and a way of life. He runs on the treadmill, he runs on the roads, he runs in marathons and has run even in the wilderness of Africa.

All of these people have experienced the 'runners high' and are much healthier and fitter for it. Running is now a passion for them, perhaps even an addiction.

WHAT IS THE RUNNER'S HIGH?

Many runners have experienced an elevated mood while running. Some have described it as a blissful state, others state it is akin to euphoria and many say that it is almost orgasmic. It may vary in degree from person to person but the runner's euphoria is felt by most regular runners. This feeling makes them forget their pains, their tiredness, their worries and their tensions and a whole new perspective of life appears.

This phenomenon may not be true for runners alone. Badminton and squash players, skiers, football players and swimmers all have their moments of high which is akin to a top-of-the-world feeling. This happens when one is performing to the maximum potential.

Though there is a debate on the exact mechanism of the runner's high, several researchers have linked the euphoria with a group of chemicals called endorphins. The word is derived from a combination of 'endogenous', meaning produced within the body and 'morphine', a narcotic derived from opium that is known for its mood alleviating and pain reduction properties. Endorphins are the body's own morphines, which give a similar feeling of exhilaration and can be enjoyed without the fear of breaking the law. This is extremely good as a stress-buster. Running, with the wind on your face and the world at your feet, leaves little scope for tensions and worries and is therefore every bit therapeutic as other forms of exercises.

OTHER BENEFITS OF RUNNING

Apart from being a stress-buster, there are many other health benefits of running which make running a great form of exercise.

Leads to a High Calorie Burn: There are very few exercises which burn more calories than running.

Fights Osteoporosis: With running, you can prevent bone and muscle loss. Running has shown an increase in the human growth hormone and so it is extremely beneficial. You can actually fight aging with running.

Prevents Diseases: Running is known to reduce the risk of stroke, heart attacks, degenerative diseases etc. Running reduces the high blood pressure levels, diabetes and raising good cholesterol. Research has shown that running boosts the immune system.

Improves Overall Health: Running helps improve overall health by reducing stress. It imparts a certain feel good factor about oneself and one's levels of confidence, self esteem etc. This could also reduce the incidence of psychosomatic illnesses.

Run for a Cure: Running is often used to treat clinical depression and other psychological disorders. Running takes away focus from the present worries and shifts it to the body, its movement and its pace. It also shifts the focus to the environment. So an individual is likely to be less tense, less depressed, less fatigued, and less confused. Studies have shown that running is a natural tranquilizer; its effects on patients with clinical depression, addictions, and disease are remarkable.

TIPS FOR STRESS-FREE RUNNING

Running is a great stress-buster, a sure shot fat burner, a fantastic mood elevator and a potent antidote against disease. But hold on, running is a double-edged sword, which can create problems if you are not careful. Since running is a high impact exercise it can potentially damage cartilage of weight bearing joints. It can raise the heart rate beyond the safety zone and cause cardiac concerns. To make running your ally a few precautions are to be taken.

Consult your Doctor before Embarking on the Running Programme
It is advisable to check your cardiac status and blood pressure with your physician and ascertain the safety limits of your running. It is also wise to wear a heart rate monitor so that you stick to the recommended heart rate zone. If you have joint problems, an orthopaedic consult will help you find out if running is allright for your joints. Certain persons with osteoarthritis and spondylosis could be better off with lesser impact exercises like cycling, swimming or walking. So it is wiser to check with a doctor before indulging in running.

Consult a Professional or a Coach
Running has a technique and one should start correctly so that bad habits do not develop. The balance, posture, stride, arm movement and foot dynamics can be set right by a running coach, who you could visit periodically to have your form assessed.

Choose a Good Surface for Running
Avoid uneven surfaces, especially those filled with potholes. Also avoid slushy and slippery grounds. Use good and appropriate footwear which can make running on hard surfaces less dangerous. If you are running in circles, it would help to alternate between clockwise and anti-clockwise routes.

Start with Low impact Exercises if you are Grossly Overweight
You could start with swimming or cycling till you reach a weight which is conducive to running. Your fitness trainer or weight loss consultant would be the person to guide you in this matter. Running with too much weight could be detrimental to the joints and could also put more strain on our heart.

Wear Good Shoes
Fantastic running shoes are available today. It is worth stretching your budget when it comes to running shoes. Ask your coach if

CHAPTER 27 : RUNNING TO DE-STRESS

your running style demands special shoes like motion control shoes or whether you need arch supports. The shoe should be well-fitting and should be changed when it loses its bounce.

Always Warm-up Before the Run and Cool down After it
Since running involves impact, the pre-run routine is very important.

Stretch Before and After the Run
Running is easier if your flexibility is optimum. The injuries are also lessened with disciplined stretching. After a warm-up you should stretch your lower extremity, back, neck and upper extremity muscles to keep them supple and in good healthy condition.

Weight Training is Helpful in giving you Better Muscles for Running
Stronger muscles, means less injury and more efficiency in running. Alternate day circuit weight training will keep the protective muscles of your knees and back strong.

Do not Over-train
Guard against overuse injury. Body awareness will teach you to respect niggles and pulls which are best rested at the first signs of showing up.

Protect against External Elements
Protect against the sun and other external elements like cold with proper attire and headgear.

Hydration and Nutrition
Hydration and nutrition are very important limbs of a running programme. Adequate water is essential and a balanced diet will help you get the best out of your run.

Subscribe to a Magazine

Subscribe to a running journal or magazine and keep abreast of the latest trends, footwear, apparel etc. to add more fun to your running schedules.

Running is a great Euphrodisiac — Baba Calm Dev

> Running gives a high like no other fitness modality. It has several health benefits and stress busting virtues, but has to be performed, keeping the precautions in mind to achieve the best results.

Swimming

CHAPTER 28

Man and water have always shared a deep romantic relationship. Water has always delighted the human senses. Whether it is just watching the deep blue sea; feeling the jacuzzi caress your back, taking the fragrance of the first rain, adding ice to your drinks, diving into the deep, crystal clear pool; hearing your opponent's golf ball landing in water...all of these immensely pleasurable sensations involve the ubiquitous water. Water is not just the elixir of life, it is also necessary for a range of necessities.

Even in the area of physical activities, water is an important element. Not only does it replace fluid, but it also is the key element in all water-based sports and entertainment zones. In fact swimming is high on the agenda for any sport lover for its potential to give the body a total work out and help keep it fit and healthy.

I started swimming in very unusual circumstances. For a short while, I attended a boarding school in Nashik, a town not far from Mumbai. An irrigation canal ran close to our school. We boys would cool off in the canal after a football game. The canal was about 15 feet wide and had chest deep easy flowing water. Many of us were not swimmers and we would just wade in, splash around and play pranks in the water.

One day as I jumped into the water, a pair of eyes looked back at me. A second later it

> Swimming is normal for me. I'm relaxed. I'm comfortable, and I know my surroundings. It's my home.
> *Michael Phelps*

was apparent that I was face to face with a snake. It was a small snake, probably a harmless water snake, but still it frightened me. In an attempt to get away from the reptile, I started splashing and kicking. When I looked up, I realized I was at the other bank. Eureka, I had swum ashore.

Fear had given me fins. It had been fight or float reaction for me!

When I returned from the boarding school, my father took great pains to see that my swimming continued. Swimming was a luxury in those days and the closest accessible pool was some twenty kilometers away from home. Still he made it a point to take me swimming every weekend.

Swimming has continued to have enthusiastic takers from our family and both my sons are proficient swimmers. A resort holiday in Sri Lanka, with lots of swimming followed by delicious food, has been a landmark vacation for our family.

Apart from swimming being great fun, it is a fabulous workout. Swimming provides you great health benefits. If on one hand, it provides the cardio benefits of running, then on the other hand, it helps you build muscle strength.

It is a great stress buster and a great way to strengthen family bonds. It is also one of the least injurious exercises.

It's hard to beat swimming when it comes to a sport that strengthens the body, soothes the mind, regulates breathing, stimulates circulation and puts no stress on the joints. Swimming is a single exercise that does it all.

Swimming is a great exercise for people who hate to sweat.

With beaches, pools and water parks accessible to the public, swimming can be part of a community fitness movement.

HEALTH BENEFITS OF SWIMMING

The list of swimming health benefits is really comprehensive.

Swimming is a popular aerobic exercise because people tend to enjoy water sports. It ensures the well-being of your heart and lungs. To ensure good cardiovascular benefits from your swimming, you need to develop a good swimming technique. A few lessons in

CHAPTER 28 : SWIMMING

swimming from a good coach are really worthwhile. A correct style of kicking and hand movements will help you glide through the water smoothly. Rhythmic breathing pattern will help you perform lap after lap with your heart rate elevated to an optimum level. According to research, just 30-60 minutes of swimming, 3-4 days per week can help reduce your risk for heart disease, stroke, and diabetes. As a regular physical activity, swimming can also help lower your blood pressure and cholesterol. The water pressure against the legs and arms is also beneficial to the circulatory system. The water pressure adds to the muscle pressure exerted on the veins to aid in returning blood to the heart and lungs.

Swimming is a great fat burner. If you can swim at a moderate pace for an hour, you could burn about 500 to 600 calories. To gain maximum fat burning benefits from swimming it is necessary to swim continuously for half an hour or more. A pulse check after few laps should confirm that you are in your aerobic training zone. Sometimes people do not achieve adequate fat loss with swimming. This is because they do not swim at the recommended intensity.

Swimming enhances the flexibility of your joints and provides the scope for boosting your physical activity workout level. A technically correct swimming stroke will help you stretch most of your upper and lower extremity muscles. As you perform the breast stroke you can help achieve a good range of movement at your shoulder, hip and knee joints.

The strength training benefits of swimming are tremendous. Water acts as resistant and a part of your body weight acts as the load. The muscles of the limbs and torso have to propel the body through the water. The muscles are given a thorough workout and one can see strength gain in a couple of weeks of swimming. Long distance swimming improves muscle endurance and sprints increase your muscle power.

Aqua-aerobics is a term for certain low impact, moderate intensity exercises performed in water. Well choreographed aqua-aerobics can help you improve your cardiovascular efficiency, burn fat, increase muscle strength and get more flexible in and outside the pool. You use a fraction of your body weight as resistance and exercise a wide range of muscles in water.

Swimming is used as a form of physical therapy for persons with musculoskeletal problems. Persons who are rehabilitating after knee surgery could do very well with a regular session in the pool.

For persons who have a hard time carrying out weight bearing physical activities on land, swimming is the answer. As the body weighs much less in water than on land, the back, knees and hips are not overstressed in the water. Swimming is just perfect for people with arthritis and back problems. Pregnant ladies can avail of swimming as a good antenatal exercise.

Swimming can be good complementary exercise to other sports. Bobby Fischer, the legendary chess player used swimming as an exercise to hone his mental skills while tackling the Russian champion, Boris Spassky. Many top golfers and tennis players use swimming as a complementary exercise to boost their primary game.

Swimming can be very relaxing and help you ward off stress. Spending time in a group, whether doing choreographed aqua-aerobics or swimming informally with friends is a great social outlet. Exchanging stories, learning new skills or strokes, or arranging mock races can make swimming a psychologically rewarding experience.

Swimming can be a form of dynamic meditation. It involves a good breathing rhythm which can induce awareness of one's being. Awareness of the breath while swimming can give you a transcendental experience where you can reach an endorphin induced state that is mood alleviating. On the other hand, lying on your back and just floating on water can give you a beautiful feeling of relaxation. This form of meditation can help you gain a feeling of well-being, leaving your water session refreshed and ready to go on with the rest of your day.

There are many more benefits of swimming apart from enhancement of health and mental relaxation. Children can derive a lot from swimming. Apart from swimming being a good exercise and a base for all round physical development, swimmers seem to do better in school. Further, swimmers develop life skills such as sportsmanship, time-management, self-discipline, goal-setting, and an increased sense of self-worth through their participation in the sport.

Swimming is an exercise which can continue to give you happiness all your life. It is immensely fulfilling. The experience of floating in water, with the nature above you, can produce a wholesome feeling that can contribute to health and happiness. It is never too late to learn the sport and once learnt, it cannot be forgotten easily. So for a lifelong, stress-busting therapy, all you need is some motivation and a swimming pool at hand.

> The list of health benefits accruing from swimming is really comprehensive. Most of the body parts are exercised effectively and safely. Flexibility, muscle strengthening, weight loss, cardio training and calmness can be achieved with swimming.

CHAPTER 29

Table Tennis

> It always pays to know your tables.
> *Baba Calm Dev*

A simple looking game, played across a net on a wooden table with a light celluloid ball, can literally uplift your spirits. I can personally vouch for the game of table tennis as being a great stress-busting medium. It has given me great joy in various stages of my life. As a kid, seeing my mother achieve great heights in the game gave me a great sense of pride. I would accompany her to many tournaments and cheer from the sidelines. It gave me a sense of pride amongst all other students in school to know that my mother was ranked 4th in the country. Partnering her in an open tournament gave me my first headline in a newspaper. My father, a university level player, played with me often and helped me hone my skills.

With good encouragement and tips from my parents I had the fortune of captaining the Bombay Schools Team and later got a chance to represent the Bombay University and the Schools combined team. Wearing the Bombay colours and playing at National level tournaments was an honour and source of ultimate happiness for me. Being a university table tennis player helped me secure additional marks to enable me get into one of the best medical colleges. Table tennis, gave me immense popularity in college. It also got me a friend like Kamlesh Mehta, India's best ever table-tennis player. As I

CHAPTER 29 : TABLE TENNIS

continue to play the game with my sons, I continue to derive immense enrichment and satisfaction in my life.

HISTORY OF TABLE TENNIS

From its humble beginning as a parlour game in England, table tennis has risen to be one of the most popular and attractive games in the world. The credit of starting table tennis possibly goes to the British officers serving in India and South Africa. It started as an indoor version of tennis where cigar box lids were used as bats, rounded wine bottle corks were used instead of balls and books substituted the net. James Gibb is credited for introducing celluloid balls and giving table tennis the name ping-pong. The term ping-pong is still used in recreational circles.

In the early part of the 20th century, the pimpled rubber bat was introduced, which remained very popular till the 1950s. The game of table tennis changed in 1952 with Hiroji Satoh of Japan introducing a wooden racket covered in thick foam sponge rubber. This racket, which produced much more speed and spin than conventional pimpled rubber rackets, revolutionized the game. Using the extra spin and speed of the sponge racket, Satoh won the 1952 World Championships beating Jozsef Koczian of Hungary. In 1970s table tennis saw a further increase in speed and spin with the use of speed glue. Dragutin Surbek of Yugoslavia discovered that using bicycle tyre repair glue to stick rubber on a blade dramatically increased the speed and spin. Lots of innovations were seen in the rubbers in the 70s, with the advent of anti spin rubbers and dead rackets. My mother, Geeta Nadkarni used a unique method to surprise her opponents by playing with a bare wooden ply on the backhand side. In 1985, the two color rule was adopted to reduce the effectiveness of combination rackets and to eliminate the surprise factor. In 1988 table tennis became an Olympic sport.

The year 2000 saw a major change in the game where the ball size and scoring patterns were changed. The diameter of the ball was increased to 40 mm and 11 point games were introduced instead of the traditional 21 points. These changes have made table tennis more popular on television. The larger ball has reduced the speed of the game, helping the camera catch the action better. The shorter 11 point game has ushered in more commercial breaks to make TT a more commercially viable and a richer sport.

BENEFITS OF TABLE TENNIS

Having enjoyed playing table tennis at a competitive level for a long time and now playing it only for recreation; I recommend this wonderful game to all, wholeheartedly. Table tennis is a fun game with a lot of health benefits where you can enhance your fitness without the risk of too many injuries.

Fitness and Health

Table tennis is a fast game which can help you raise your heart rate. TT can give you a good aerobic workout, where in you can burn fat and improve your heart function. You do not have to be a professional to get the best out of TT. Even a recreational player can work up a good sweat and improve general fitness and health.

Easy on Your Body

Being a non-contact sport, there are very few injuries associated with table tennis. If one warms up and stretches before a game, the injuries are further minimized. A person with back problems, however needs to be careful as there is some amount of back flexion required to play the game effectively.

Everyone Can Play

Like all other games, there is no age or gender limits when it comes to playing table tennis. I have played in club tournaments where there are events like jumbled doubles. In jumbled doubles lots are drawn and 60 year old veterans often play with 15 year old juniors or have men playing against women. Everyone has a great time with lots of cheering and bonhomie.

Like golf, table tennis is a lifelong sport. TT can be played right up to your seventies and beyond. It's never too late to start and there is no retirement age! Since the game is gentle on the body, veterans too can play competitively and enjoy the game. Better technology like super fast or anti-spin rubbers can compensate for age-related slowing reflexes.

Table Tennis Meditation
Table tennis can also send you into a transcendental zone. Long rallies at a fast pace in TT have sent me into a meditative state many times. The ball is hit almost reflexively and you are soon in the moment. There is no scope for worry or tension, as the game itself grips you.

Anytime, Anyplace Game
Being a non-seasonal indoor game, table tennis can be played all the year round. Be it day or night, TT can always be played. You don't need protection from the sun or rain or snow. Schools, colleges, clubs and hotels find it convenient to house a few tables, making the game even more popular. Since the space required is not too much, table tennis can be played even at home. Most tables can be folded and kept away after the game.

Make Friends for Life
Since this is a game that involves inter-personal interaction, so it does provide ground for increasing your social life. Industrialist Niraj Bajaj, a former national TT champion has an annual get-together of ex-state players at his house. The camaraderie and the bonding among the players is to be seen to be believed. Social status or age does not come between friends who have played this great game together. I have been lucky to have played this game with some wonderful people, who are friends for life.

Not Expensive
You don't have to spend a fortune to play table tennis. The equipment consisting of a racket, balls and shoes is most affordable. Compared to golf and tennis, the membership costs to TT clubs are

often quite low, contributing to its popularity.

If you are looking for an inexpensive, enjoyable, injury free, fitness enhancing, stress buster of a game; then Table Tennis is the right sport for you. It's a total work out minus stress, strain and injury and keeps worries at bay.

> If you are looking for an inexpensive, enjoyable, injury free, fitness enhancing, stress buster of a game, then it is table tennis. If you play the game with some consistency, the meditative aspect of table tennis can be enjoyed.

CHAPTER 30

Golf

Golf is intimately connected to Calm Sutra. Golf played with concentration can produce a state much like nirvana. This is because of the awareness of experience that it involves. Awareness transports you to nirvana. When you swing the club smoothly and hit the ball with the sweet spot of your club-head, a unique sensation is experienced. This sensation is multiplied as you see the ball in flight and go the distance. Nothing else exists. You are in the moment and that unique sensation is in you.

It was in May 1992 that my life changed. I was pretty normal at that time. That was before we went to Munnar, for our summer vacation. Munnar is the scenic capital of Gods own land, Kerala. We were staying at the High Range Club, a great souvenir of the British Raj. The club is housed in the midst of lush green, manicured tea gardens. The club has its lounge with a piano, a fire place and heads of bison looking down at you. It has a men's only bar, a snooker room, a library and of course a golf course. The club has kept up its English traditions, with jacket and ties for evenings, games of tambola and jam sessions. The club also has a tennis court, which was well utilized by our family till that fateful day.

I remember that fateful day very well. I was playing tennis with my nephew, when it started raining. It was unseasonal rain and we thought it would stop. The rain went on to

> Golf is both ballistic and holistic.
> *Baba Calm Dev*

CALM SUTRA : THE ART OF RELAXATION

drench the clay court and soon it became unplayable. As we were trudging back, unhappily towards the club house, a young boy walked up to us. How can I forget his face and his smile?

'Play golf, Sir?' he asked. 'Golf and me', I laughed and said, 'Golf is for the old fogies, with no athletic prowess or skill to play any other decent game. What kind of a game is it where you need a servant to carry your equipment?'

He smiled and said, 'Sir, you have good body. You will hit long ball.' He was advocating a foolish game, but the young lad had an eye to identify a good physique and surely he could notice my exceptional ball sense! I took up his bait.

Soon I found myself on the first tee, with Manikandan, yes that was his name, handing me a long stick with a wooden head. My only exposure to golf was seeing Nick Faldo and Greg Norman striding the greens on TV, while flipping channels. Manikandan teed up a ball and pointed in the direction of a red flag far away. 'Hit Sir', he said.

I held the stick, like what resembled a baseball grip, and swung it with all my might. This is where beginners luck and destiny conspired to lure me away from normalcy. The ball I hit took off like a supersonic jet, went more than 200 meters and came to rest in the middle of the fairway. The shot gave me the pleasure of a hundred cross court backhands and several tennis service aces. I had been consumed by the game.

With great pride and the swagger of a professional golfer, I ambled down the fairway. Manikandan held a stick with a metal end this time. The flag, he said was a hundred meters away and that a nine iron would take my ball to it. With my son Nishad and nephews as audience I took an almighty swing. We tried looking for the ball flying towards the flag, but no luck. The ball had not moved a millimeter. I had missed the ball by six inches. I had managed to dig a crater into the beautiful ground, with so much force that it could have registered a tremor on the Richter's scale. In the next few shots I had managed to kill a few earthworms, scare some squirrels out of their trees and change the hibernation

CHAPTER 30 : GOLF

clocks of other animals. In trying to come out of the bunkers, I had gathered much sand on me, making Lawrence of Arabia look like a freshly bathed baby. The game stopped only after I had managed to lose all of Manikandan's balls. The game of golf had dented my ego. But I was not a quitter. I wanted to prove that the first shot was not a fluke. And I came back to the course, the next day, to salvage my pride. That's how golf crept into my life, at the expense of normalcy.

WHAT IS GOLF?

Says Arnold Palmer, one of the legends in golfing history: "Golf is deceptively simple and endlessly complicated; it satisfies the soul and frustrates the intellect. It is at the same time rewarding and maddening - and it is without a doubt the greatest game mankind has ever invented."

Trying to explain golf to the uninitiated, in terms of difficulty, ranks second to explaining cricket to an American. It is a challenging task but I will try. The basic idea in golf is to hit a ball, with a club, from a tee, into a hole, in the least number of strokes. The distance from the tee to the hole may vary from a mere hundred odd meters to over 500 meters. A par three hole demands that you hole the ball in 3 shots, a par four in 4 and a par five in 5 shots. You first hit a long shot off the tee, approach the hole with some accurate shots and then putt the ball in the hole. If you manage to hole a par four hole in 4 shots and I hole it in 5, you win the hole.

The golf equipment consists of a set of 14 clubs or sticks. The game is played on a golf course usually of 18 holes. It is one game you can play alone, but is often played in pairs, as a threesome and most commonly as a four-ball. You usually walk more than 6 kilometers as you finish 18 holes. The game is full of golfing terms like pars, birdies, bogeys, handicaps etc., which can best be understood when you start playing the game. The game may sound simple to play considering you are hitting a stationary ball, but the unpredictability in golf makes the game exciting and addictive. In fact golf is a huge leveler. It can make a professional play like an amateur on one day and an amateur play like a professional on another day. So it does cut down on egos and pride.

BENEFITS OF GOLF

There are great benefits to be had from golf. The body, mind, soul and probably even the social stature, business contacts etc. all stand to gain on the golf course. These days, most of the high flying deals are being made on the golf course as it it is the place top notch businessmen and corporate honchos frequently go to and combine business with pleasure.

At a certain level, golf and meditation are akin to each other and have thus been termed soul mates. Each one complements the other. Golf is about style, panache, concentration, strength, tenacity, keen eye and a brilliant sense of judgement. However, more than anything else, this game is about patience, absolute and heightened. So it is with meditation making them complete partners or soul mates. Golf with its deep history and tradition is a wholesome form of stress busting exercise and contributes to the all round development of the player.

Fat Loss

Golf involves walking, unless it is a buggy course. So it can be very effective for losing calories. In fact almost all the benefits of walking can be derived here since golf involves a fair amount of walking.

Cardiovascular Exercise

Golf can also help in getting benefits of aerobic exercises especially if one carries golf bag or at least pulls a trolley. The added burden of the golf clubs can give a good workout to the heart-lung complex. I have played at some hilly courses like the ones in Ooty and Wellington which act like stress test machines. The pulse rate can be kept in a good zone if you are playing as a twosome and walk fast.

Muscle Flexibility

The game of golf is played with the entire body and not just with the arms. The muscles of the back, torso and the upper extremities are stretched during a good golf swing. The stretching and pre-game loosening exercise ensure good flexibility in the muscles used in golf.

Muscle Strength

The modern professional golfer is a fit, strong person hitting the ball over mammoth distances. Even the recreational golfer taking cue from the professional, indulges in some strength training exercises through the week to be a stronger hitter. Light weight training designed for the golfing muscles can increase the muscle power and endurance and keep injuries at bay.

Mental Agility

Golf offers a mental challenge. You're always thinking while on the golf course, whether it's counting your opponent's shots, or calculating yardages for club selection or planning on the next shot. All that mental exercise is good for you. It is especially effective for those who are in the older age group as it keeps the brain active and prevents the incidence of Alzheimer's disease.

Sunshine and Greenery

Golf is one opportunity to be in green surroundings away from the pollution, and noise. The green expanses are soothing to the eye as well as to the other senses. Being on the golf course is mentally relaxing and being in the game is mentally stimulating. Also the air and the sunshine provide benefits to the bone and muscle formation. Hence golf is a great boost for the senses. For a doctor who spends most of the day in air-conditioned clinics and operation theatres, the golf course is a great place for me to soak in the sunshine, which can work wonders on the bones as well as the psyche.

Meditation

When you swing the golf club or are putting with great concentration everything else is pushed to the background. Golf can create a doorway to nirvana. Conversely meditation techniques help the golf game tremendously, by slowing down the thoughts and facilitating an easy, smooth swing.

Manners and Etiquettes

Tiger Woods has come up with a foundation called 'The First Tee' which teaches children golf. It also teaches them core values like courtesy, honesty, integrity, respect, responsibility etc. which help them become better citizens. A child who has grown up on the golf course usually develops good values which are consistent with the game of golf.

Friends

The biggest bonus golf has given me is 'friends'. After the school and college days the new group of friends, I have made, is on the golf course. Friendship made on the golf course often extends beyond the greens. It manifests in the hospital when someone is sick, it emerges when someone needs help in business, it celebrates anniversaries and birthdays, goes on vacations together; but somehow it disappears when it comes to giving putts on the green! That's the time friends become rivals, pitting their mental and physical prowess against each other. This is what pushes stress in the back seat and helps develop a strong and mentally agile personality that is able to handle the vagaries of life rather adeptly.

Recently I have seen friendship being taken to a different level by my dear friend and co-golfer, Kishore Musale. Kishore is an avid golfer who seeks refuge in work during the week, to try and forget his losses in golf over the weekend. And his work speaks for itself. He is emerging as a force to reckon with, on the Indian industrial scene. After a Sunday golf round, we demanded a party from him for his outstanding achievements. He nodded vaguely. Next we receive a message from his office asking for our passports. The

CHAPTER 30 : GOLF

tickets are couriered and soon Kishore and 8 of his friends are off to South Africa. Yes Kishore hosted his party on the fabulous golf courses of Durban and Cape Town.

GETTING STARTED

There is no substitute for golf lessons from qualified professionals and that is the only way to learn golfing techniques the right way. I started the game accidentally, with Manikandan as my coach. Though I am thankful to Manikandan for giving me the taste of golf, I am sure my game would have been better off had I taken lessons from a proper coach. The habits you develop early in golf remain with you. As for me, I have a bit of cricket, tennis and table-tennis in my golf swing. Though my swing does not resemble the action of a snake slayer or a folk dancer from Gujarat, it is far from perfect.

A good golf teacher will teach you the correct grip, stance, body alignment, swing and follow through. The correct swing will not only help you play better, it will minimize the chances of injury. A bad swing can have far-reaching consequences on your back. A tight awkward grip can lead to conditions like a golfer's elbow. An ergonomically enhanced swing, taught by a good coach will be smooth and balanced, and which will involve the use of the entire body rather than just the arms. With a good transfer of body weight into the ball, you are more likely to hit the ball at the right pace and length and therefore enjoy success in this beautiful game for a long time.

The game of golf also requires some basic fitness and a sound pre-game routine for enhanced success. Stretching exercises are essential to maintain good flexibility. Some amount of light weight training will help you gain strength and improve your ball striking. A basic cardio exercise like cycling or treadmill walking will increase your stamina and decrease the fatigue factor during your golf round. A good pre-game routine of warm up and loosening exercises are mandatory. A few practice swings or a short session

CALM SUTRA : THE ART OF RELAXATION

on the driving range before the round, will not only improve your game, but also reduce the chances of injury.

Golf is considered by many to an upper class indulgence. These days, the number of corporates calling the shots on the greens is swelling. Golf is currently on the way to establishing itself as a 'corporate' game mainly because of its stress busting properties in a visually appealing ambience. Golf hones almost all skills that are required for high pressure jobs; skills like concentration, analysis, patience, restructuring strategies, following opposing trends etc. This is what is making the corporate sector push the 'golf agenda'.

Therefore, rush to the greens and grab your moment on it. Acquire a membership to a golf club or become a member of your local golf union and just tee off towards happiness and health.

Golf benefits the body, mind and soul. Walking in beautiful surroundings with total body swings helps you remain healthy and fit. Playing the game mindfully and with full awareness makes golf a form of Green Meditation. The quality time you spend with friends, adds another dimension to your life.

Epilogue

I hope you have enjoyed reading the *Calm Sutra*, just as I have enjoyed writing it.

The crux of the *Calm Sutra* can be summarized in two words, Awareness and Action.

Awareness, practiced in life, can usher in a state of calm and tranquility.

Awareness of body posture, breathing and thought enables us to live in the moment. Living in the moment usually allows us to have a hold on our thoughts and actions and imparts a strength that eliminates worry and stress.

Awareness influences good Action.

Awareness of body posture translates to Action, creating better posture.

Awareness of breath leads to Action, influencing deeper and slower breathing.

Awareness of thought gives birth to the Meditation.

Awareness of thought also gives us a chance to take a Calm Pause. This Calm Pause helps us gather meandering thoughts and streamlines the same so as to form a favorable proactive response for stress.

Awareness of tension results in Relaxation.

Action with Awareness makes the Action transcendental.

Actions as described in the *Calm Sutra*, like walking, swimming, singing, dancing and exercising when performed with Awareness makes the action meditative.

Action with Awareness in golf enables you to hit the ball straight and far... towards success.

The Calm Sutra Workshop (CSW)

Dr Dilip Nadkarni conducts interactive workshops on *Calm Sutra: The Art of Relaxation* for Corporate audiences.

The Calm Sutra Workshop (CSW)is a practical training programme where most stress-busters described in the book are discussed, demonstrated and practiced.

CSW will help you increase your AWARENESS of thought, breath and posture.

The ACTION at CSW includes learning techniques like deep breathing, meditation, visualization, affirmation and progressive muscle relaxation.

Simple fitness enhancing exercises and postural tips are provided to improve health and reduce degenerative conditions.

Dr. Dilip Nadkarni is an acknowledged entertrainer par excellence and the sessions are filled with laughter, music and dance.

CSW will energize you and yet help you be calm. It will enhance your performance as you learn to manage stress and be happy.

CSW is guaranteed to change your life!

www.calmsutra.org

About the Author

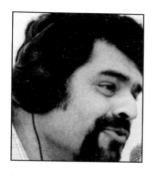

Dr. Dilip Nadkarni is an orthopaedic surgeon specializing in treating sports and fitness-related injuries. He is a distinction holder in MBBS and a gold medalist in post-graduation in orthopaedic surgery from Mumbai, India. He treats top international sportspersons and filmstars engaged in fitness activity.

Dr. Nadkarni is attached to Lilavati Hospital in Mumbai, where he performs advanced arthroscopic surgery. He has written a book titled *Knee Problem... No Problem*, which deals with avoiding and coping with knee disorders. He also edits a website called www.kneecure.com.

Dr. Nadkarni's another book titled *REAL Fitness* gives a simple formula to fitness, which includes relaxation, exercise, attitude and laughter. He launched the "Fit India Movement" to promote fitness and give lectures on TV, radio, sports clubs, Rotary clubs, Lions clubs, social organizations and corporate bodies. He has scripted and produced an instructional fitness video "Fitness Forever".

After conducting several workshops on stress management involving meditation, music, visualization and golf, in India and abroad, Dr. Nadkarni has written *Calm Sutra*. With *Calm Sutra*, he gives a formula for a healthy, happy and stress-free living. Dr Nadkarni hosts an interactive website, www.calmsutra.org

He has played table tennis at the national level and now plays amateur golf. He is a songwriter as well as a music composer with original works to his credit.

Dr. Dilip Nadkarni lives in Mumbai with his wife Rashmi, an anaesthesiologist, and his sons Nishad and Rishab.